Ayurvedic
Healing Cuisine

Other books by Harish Johari:

Attunements for Dawn and Dusk (CD)
Ayurvedic Massage
The Birth of the Ganga
Breath, Mind, and Consciousness
Chakras
Chants to the Sun and Moon
Dhanwantari
The Healing Power of Gemstones
Leela
The Monkeys and the Mango Tree
Numerology
The Planet Meditation Kit
Sounds of Tantra (audiocassette)
Sounds of the Chakras (audiocassette)
Tools for Tantra

Ayurvedic
Healing Cuisine

200 Vegetarian Recipes
for Health, Balance,
and Longevity

Harish Johari

Healing Arts Press
Rochester, Vermont

Healing Arts Press
One Park Street
Rochester, Vermont 05767
www.InnerTraditions.com

Healing Arts Press is a division of Inner Traditions International

*Note to the reader. This book is intended as an informational guide The remedies, approaches, and techniques
described herein are meant to supplement, and not to be a substitute for, professional medical care or treatment
They should not be used to treat a serious ailment without prior consultation with a qualified health care professional*

Library of Congress Cataloging-in-Publication Data

Johari, Harish, 1934–1999.
    [Healing Cuisine]
    Ayurvedic healing cuisine : 200 vegetarian recipes for health, balance, and
longevity / Harish Johari.
        p. cm.
    Previously published: Healing cuisine. 1994.
    Includes index.
    ISBN 0-89281-938-3 (alk. paper)
    1. Vegetarian cookery. 2. Medicine, Ayurvedic. 3. Indian cookery. I. Title.

RM236 .J64 2000
613 2'62—dc21

                                                    00-040914

Printed and bound in Canada at Transcontinental

10 9 8 7 6 5 4

Text design and layout by Charlotte Tyler
This book was typeset in Weiss

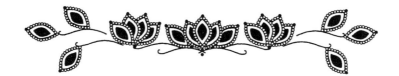

CONTENTS

→ Appendices ←

EDITOR'S NOTE

The first manuscript to come to Inner Traditions (Healing Arts Press) from Harish Johari was *The Healing Cuisine*. It was a massive five hundred pages, painstakingly hand-written and containing a wealth of Ayurvedic cooking knowledge and recipes here-tofore unavailable in the West. That was more than ten years ago. In the interim, we have published six other titles by Harish (and three audiocassettes). Why did it take us so long to publish this title, especially as we received frequent calls and letters from Harish's friends from all over this country and abroad in search of the finished book?

To watch Harish preparing a meal—whether for four or for twenty-four—is to watch a master at work. Completely attentive to the task at hand, he cooks with every one of his senses. His hands, seemingly under invisible, inaudible instruction, simply know what to do. People are inevitably drawn into the kitchen to watch or to participate. There is always learning going on (Harish is, after all, a teacher of the first order) and a good bit of laughter. If you are willing, he will put you to work chopping vegetables or making chapatis. And while nothing overtly extraordinary is happening, a good deal of time goes by, a great deal of knowledge is passed along, and the result is always the sharing of an extraordinary meal.

It is hard to translate this experience into print. All the recipes were written in a manner consistent with Harish's cooking style—charming, intuitive, and intelligible only if you were lucky enough to be at his elbow. The manuscript was put on hold for a couple of years while we mustered our courage. Finally, Harish and our editors set about the long process of translating the original text into a language and format that could be used by any cook in his or her Western kitchen (with the addition of some ingredients and implements that are described in the book).

The tradition of apprenticeship has, sadly, fallen away in many of our endeavors, but it is very much alive in the pages of this book. May the learning and laughter of that tradition be mixed in equal measure with the healing principles of Ayurvedic cooking.

—Leslie Colket Blair

INTRODUCTION

Health is the state of harmonious chemical balance in a living organism. Our health depends on the chemical environments inside and outside our bodies. Food plays an important role in creating the internal chemical environment. Cooking food makes it palatable, digestible, and assimilable.

When cooked properly, food is appetizing, flavorful, and aromatic. Cooking is a way of offering love. Food that is cooked with love, guided by knowledge of the ingredients being cooked, and served in an inspiring atmosphere becomes healing. Food is something very personal and it should never be eaten for taste alone; its purpose is to provide nutrients and satisfaction to the body, without introducing toxins. This satisfaction comes from a state of electrochemical balance inside the organism, which is created by the postdigestive action of the food. A major part of chemical imbalance is created by living with incorrect habits and in a bad environment. This situation can be counteracted by eating good, healthful food.

Vegetarian food cooked with healing herbs and energizing spices can eliminate many of the toxins that have entered the body through polluted water and air, or even noise. Toxins also enter us through radiation or chemicals that are supposed to prevent our food from decay and that are used freely on vegetables, fruits, and all types of edible foodstuffs. Spices—concentrated "chemicals" that are converted into cleansing and vitalizing frequencies by our electrochemical system—save our body from chemical imbalance.

Cooking therefore is an art and a science at the same time. It is an art when the cook is inspired and completely absorbed in inventing a new dish, a new taste. When the cook, like a medicine man, uses herbs and spices to enhance the nutritional value, cooking is a science. But when the art and science of cooking combine in a cook, cooking becomes alchemy and food becomes Tantra. The love of the cook rejuvenates each and every cell of the body and food becomes an elixir, a tonic, a vitalizer, and a medicine.

A good cook knows that taste is a key to the chemical nature of food and that through taste he or she can manipulate the chemical environment of the body. There are six tastes and six kinds of taste buds; good food satisfies all the taste buds. A cook who knows the Ayurvedic principles of taste— for example, that the sweet taste is a combination of water and earth elements and it subdues *Vata* (Wind) and *Pitta* (Bile) and stimulates *Kapha* (Mucus)—can play with these tastes and subdue the aggravated humor to reestablish the chemical balance.

Cooking is a way of caring that gives complete satisfaction. Indian cooks derive their knowledge of herbs and spices, vegetables, legumes, and so forth from Ayurveda, which helps them maintain physical, mental, social, and spiritual harmony.

A good cook should remember that alkaline body chemistry is an important key to good health and a long life. All foods should create such a balance that the body chemistry is predominantly alkaline. With age, body chemistry becomes more acidic and the wear-and-tear mechanism becomes more powerful. If older people introduce alkaline foods or foods whose postdigestive action is alkaline into their diets, they can remain healthy and live long lives.

The philosophy, cooking methods, and recipes in this book are based on Ayurveda, the most ancient system of Indian medicine. Ayurveda studies the physical and psychic behavior of people and prescribes ways for them to synchronize with their environment so as to live happy, healthy, and inspired lives.

Much emphasis is given to diet, following the cycles of the seasons, getting up before dawn, massage, and other useful practices for enriching life.

Information dealing with diseases, their diagnosis, and cures also exists within Ayurveda. It even encompasses surgery and plastic surgery.* The term "Ayurveda" comes from *ayu* meaning "life" and *veda* meaning "knowledge." The Greek system of medicine, which is parallel to Ayurveda, is called "Unani-Tib"—*Unani* meaning "Greek" and *tib*, "medicine." These two medical systems understand and define the body in similar ways, and each incorporates the principles of *doshas* (humors), pulse, and diet. While it is hard to say whether they both stem from the same source, in India both Ayurveda and Unani-Tib are practiced.

---

*Majno, Guido. *The Healing Hand: Man and Wound in the Ancient World.* Cambridge: Harvard University Press, 1975.

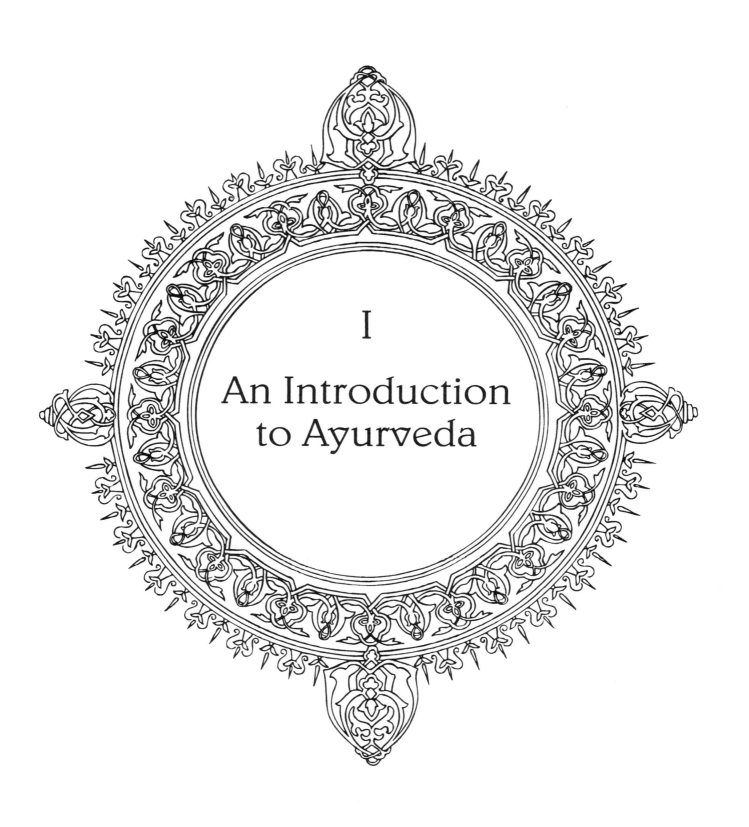

I

An Introduction to Ayurveda

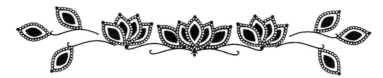

Chapter One

PRINCIPLES OF AYURVEDA

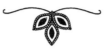

THE FIVE ELEMENTS

All phenomenal existence is an interplay of different frequencies of vibrations, from the most subtle to the most dense. Ayurvedic seers and sages have classified these vibrations into a system of five elements. These elements are agents of the primary inertia principle of consciousness and belong to the material field. They are the materialized form of the universal energy, which exists as a continuum of frequencies.

Akasha, or ether, evolved first and is the most subtle of the five elements. From it comes air, from air evolves fire, from fire comes water, and from water comes earth. The human body, which is composed of these elements, is also nourished and maintained by them. They are responsible for all its psychophysical properties. In the body the five elements assume the form of the three doshas and work with the chemical nature of the organism. The three doshas are in fact the physiological counterparts of the five elements: Akasha and air combine to create the humor of Vata; air and fire combine to create the humor of Pitta; water and earth combine to produce the humor of Kapha.

THE TRIDOSHA THEORY

According to Ayurveda, the three humors or doshas—Vata (Wind), Pitta (Bile), and Kapha (Mu-

cus)—are responsible for the functioning of the human organism. When these three doshas reside undisturbed in their proper places—that is, in specific organs and tissues—the organism is supported by them and is in balance. When disturbed, they cause disease and deterioration of the body.

Of all the doshas, Wind is the key. Bile and Mucus cannot move from their centers unless the air within the body carries them. If just one of these three doshas is disturbed, the diseases produced are easily curable. Diseases produced by the disturbance of two doshas become comparatively chronic and require more time to heal. When diseases are caused by the disorder of all three, the condition often becomes fatal.

INDIVIDUAL TEMPERAMENTS

These three doshas produce various temperaments and physical types, depending on their proportion in an individual. The rhythmic pattern of these humors fluctuates periodically, since the doshas are affected by place, climate, change of season, diet, and a score of other factors; the individual temperament, however, remains the same.

Some people are clearly dominated by one of the three doshas, while others are dominated by various combinations. Of the seven categories listed below, the first three are basic: Wind-dominated (Vata), Bile-dominated (Pitta), Mucus-dominated

(Kapha); Wind- and Bile-dominated (Vata and Pitta), Wind- and Mucus-dominated (Vata and Kapha), Bile- and Mucus-dominated (Pitta and Kapha), and Wind-, Bile-, and Mucus-dominated (Vata and Pitta and Kapha, in equal proportion).

Wind-dominated Individuals (Vatas)*

The term *vata* comes from the Sanskrit *va*, which means "to move." Wind-dominated individuals are prone to sleeplessness and dislike the cold and things that are cold. The slightest exposure to cold gives them pain in the body. The skin of such persons is dry; their hair is thin, sparse, and brittle. They have a restless mind and a weak memory. These people are often constipated, they yawn a lot, and their mouths are frequently dry. They are sometimes very hungry, while other times they are not hungry at all. They like sweet-, sour-, and salty-tasting foods. They are lovers of sexual and sensual enjoyment but do not have many offspring. They stammer when they speak. In their dreams, they dwell on mountains, in trees, and in the air; they dream of flying without mechanical aids. These people are tall and thin. Although strongly built, in reality they are weak. Hot and unctuous foods are suitable for them.

Bile-dominated Individuals (Pittas)

The term *pitta* comes from the Sanskrit word *tap*, which translates as "to produce heat." Bile-dominated individuals are angry in disposition, and they sweat profusely. They are learned, brave, and proud. They are lovers of flowers and aromatic scents. Such persons have a holy outlook and are self-supported, kind, and courageous. They do not follow the prevalent religions. Their face and eyes have a reddish cast, their body temperatures are hot, and they are quick-tempered and easily excitable. Often hungry and thirsty, they are lovers of sweet, bitter, and astringent tastes, and are fond of cold drinks and cold climates. Pittas eat a great deal and have a tendency toward obesity. They are jealous in nature. They go to the bathroom frequently. They have loose joints and muscles, and moderate-to-weak sexual desire. They avoid disturbances. In dreams, they see stars, fire, the sun, the moon, lightning, shining objects, and poisonous plants. Cold, heavy, and dry foods are suitable for this type of temperament.

Mucus-dominated Individuals (Kaphas)

Kapha comes from the Sanskrit term *shlish*, which means "to join, embrace, or adhere." Mucus-dominated individuals are handsome, well-built, symmetrical, and possess ample fat reserves. Sober and forgiving in nature, they have stable and steady minds and are religiously inclined. The face of a mucus-dominated person is moonlike; their skin color is like brass, gold, or a lotus flower. Such persons have attractive, broad foreheads; their hair is dense and strong. They are not disturbed by hunger, thirst, or noise. They have noble qualities, are sweet-spoken, fond of order, and honor their own words. They have good digestion, eat moderately, and enjoy good health. Lovers of sexual enjoyment, they have many children and loyal friends. They spend a great deal of time in thought and take time to complete tasks. They are shy and devoted to their teachers. They like bitter-, astringent-, and pungent-tasting foods. They sleep a lot and experience sound sleep. They enjoy fine arts. The dreams of such people are about rivers, ponds, oceans, lakes, and water birds. Mucus-dominated people (Kaphas) are susceptible to coughs and colds. Hot, light, and dry foods are suitable for this type of temperament.

One should remember that all of the qualities described are not present at once in someone belonging to one of these categories. By carefully observing oneself and by noting the actions of particular foods on one's system, the exact temperament, or temperament combinations, may be diagnosed. In general, Ayurveda advises eating foods that balance the intrinsic characteristics of the dominant dosha, rather than increasing (aggravating) the existing condition.

DHATUS

The word *dhatu* is derived from *dha*, "to put or place." Because the dhatus put the body in a form, or con-

---

*While the correct plural form is Vataja, Pittaja, and Kaphaja, for simplicity we are just adding an "s."

struct it, they are known as the root principles or elemental constituents of the body. There are seven dhatus:

1. *Rasa* (plasma) derived from the essence of food.
2. *Rakta* (blood) derived from the essence of rasa.
3. *Mamsa* (flesh) derived from the essence of rakta.
4. *Meda* (fat) derived from the essence of mamsa.
5. *Asthi* (bones) derived from the essence of meda.
6. *Majja* (marrow) derived from the essence of asthi.
7. *Shukra* (semen) derived from the essence of majja.

Rasa provides nourishment; Rakta, vitality; Mamsa, strength; Meda, reserve energy; Asthi, support; Majja, viscidity; Shukra, satisfaction. Together they are responsible for growth and maintenance of the body. Dhatus are influenced by doshas. Doshas are the active principles that influence the chemical environment inside the body. When the doshas are deranged, they influence the dhatus and create disease. When the body is in proper balance, doshas carry nourishment and help in cleaning the various systems of the body. The nourishment is accepted by the dhatus and whatever is not acceptable is discharged from the body, with the help of the doshas.

THE THREE DOSHAS

Wind, Bile, and Mucus represent respectively the aerial, fiery, and liquid forms of life energy, wherever they may manifest themselves in the organism. It should be understood that the three doshas regulate and balance the human organism. Each dosha has its own part to play in the maintenance of the body.

Wind

Wind is swift, dry, light, cool, and possessed of motion. This dosha is formed of the elements air and ether (akasha). Wind is the primary principle of movement in the body. It changes its nature according to changes in temperature and pressure. Wind transports whatever it comes into contact with. If it flows over a garden full of fragrant flowers, it carries the scent of the flowers. By moving along its own interior vessels, Wind affects the unobstructed functioning of the processes of the vascular, digestive, and nervous systems. All movements, whether conscious or unconscious, are performed with the

help of Wind. It is Wind that provides pneumatic power to the hydraulic pumps of the vascular and lymphatic systems. While it flows throughout the body, the main abodes of the Wind humor are the hips and the colon.

Although Wind, or *Vayu*, is unified in nature, depending on the location and nature of its movement, it is divided into five subcategories: Prana, Udana, Samana, Vyana, Apana.

Prana Vata. Prana Vayu, or Prana Vata, located in the region of the chest, is the air in the body. It is of primary importance for it is the air one breathes and the air that helps in swallowing, spitting, sneezing, chewing, and maintaining the action of the heart, mind, and senses. Prana also provides nourishment to the lungs and the heart. Beginning in the head, Prana makes its way to the mouth, coordinating muscular movements of the tongue, throat, and cheek before going on to the thoracic region. Prana Vata is the air of the heart chakra. In the practice of certain yogic techniques, such as *pranayama*, meditation, Nada Yoga, or Swara Yoga, it helps in raising the energy to the crown of the head. Prana works with the sympathetic and parasympathetic nervous systems and produces psychic currents. The word *prana* in Sanskrit is synonymous with life. This is considered the most important of the five subcategories of the Wind dosha.

Udana Vata. Udana is located in the thoracic and throat regions It extends from the upper part of the stomach to the top of the cranium. It is Udana Vata that produces various sounds and facilitates the phenomenon of speech. Udana Vata vibrates the nasal passages and the cranium when a person hums.

Samana Vata. Samana resides between the region of the heart and the navel. It extends the length of the ascending colon and into the descending colon, circulating in the stomach and small intestine. With the help of digestive juices in the stomach, Samana changes the chemical nature of food and separates nutrients from waste materials. Samana gives physical strength to the body.

Vyana Vata. Located in the heart, this body air circulates continuously through the whole body. Vyana Vata flows through the blood vessels as the blood gases and through the lymphatic and nervous systems. It provides nourishment from one part of the body to the other; making the blood flow, it causes sweating and cleanses the body of toxins. Movements of all kinds—getting up, sitting down, pushing, pulling, opening the eyes—are all done by Vyana. It works with the central, sympathetic, and parasympathetic nervous systems.

Apana Vata. Apana, located in the pelvic region, expels the toxins accumulated in this region. These toxins can destroy digestive fire and create illness. Apana Vata also facilitates both the contraction of the uterus at orgasm and the holding of the conceived child in the womb. It helps in urination, the discharge of menstrual fluid, the delivery of a child, and the ejaculation of seminal fluid. Apana Vata plays an important role in the preservation of the human species.

Bile

As the representative of the fire and water elements, Bile is hot, fiery, wet, and fetid. In the same way that Wind controls movement, this dosha controls metabolism. Dark yellow in color, bile turns bluish-yellow when mixed with mucus. Bile provides body heat and thus provides inspiration and incentive to struggle for and achieve the objects of desire. Bile is sharp in taste (like chili pepper), moist, greasy, and has a smooth consistency. Its main abode is the upper intestine. Bile functions to "cook" and mature foods. It extracts the energies of foods in the form of fluids and causes these energies to be radiated throughout the body. Bile induces hunger and thirst and provides powers of determination, discrimination, and intellectualization to the brain.

Bile, or Pitta, is divided into five subcategories, based on function: Pachaka, Ranjaka, Sadhaka, Alochaka, and Bhrajaka. Each is fed from the main storehouse in the abdomen.

Pachaka Pitta means "digestive." Produced in the liver and pancreas, Pachaka Pitta increases digestive fire in the upper digestive tract. It chemically separates the nutritional essence from the solid and liquid wastes, and separates Wind and Mucus. Pachaka Pitta, through its fire, eliminates toxins and poisons contained in food. It helps in the production of antibodies, which are the saviors of the body. Pachaka Pitta is the main Bile, the one upon which the other four subcategories depend.

Ranjaka Pitta, or "reddening" bile, is the secretion of the liver and spleen. When nutrients reach the liver and spleen, they react with Ranjaka. The chemical reaction that takes place converts the nutrients into a form that is directly assimilable by the bloodstream, creating the red color of the blood. Through this reaction the bile is converted into a substance that can be directly assimilated into the bloodstream. What remains of the Ranjaka Pitta is utilized in digesting food.

Sadhaka Pitta, located in the heart, is responsible for maintaining the balance of oxygen and glucose. It provides inspiration, courage, and determination—the most important requirements for self-realization and growth. *Sadhaka* means "beholder." This type of bile gives one the power to pursue spiritual desires and longings and is thus helpful for spiritual aspirants. For all religious practices, inspiration, courage, perseverance, and determination are needed. These qualities exist only when a proper mixture of oxygen and glucose is present in the bloodstream. If the glucose content is low, nervousness is experienced. If the glucose supply is stable, then one feels great courage and inspiration. Sadhaka Pitta also serves as an aid to memory, the capacity to understand, the determinative intellect, and the attainment of spiritual bliss—the state of *samadhi.*

Alochaka Pitta refers to the bile that resides in the eyes. It is the fiery energy that fixes the colors and shapes of the objects that we see. This form of bile balances the heat in the eye tissues and in the muscles that control and regulate light input.

Bhrajaka Pitta means "shining." This type of bile, located in the skin, provides a healthy glow (*ojas*) to the skin and to all internal organs. Bhrajaka Pitta digests oil massaged into the skin. It nourishes and lubricates the skin, produces luster and a good complexion, and protects the body against germs. This bile also reacts to atmospheric conditions and interacts with the electromagnetic field of the earth. Bhrajaka Pitta is distributed throughout the body. However, when any psychophysical problem arises, it is withdrawn; with its withdrawal, the glow of the skin departs.

Mucus

Mucus is a mixture of the water and earth elements. This dosha controls structure. Mucus is white, heavy, smooth, cold, sticky, sweet, and fluid. It is found throughout the body. Mucus is responsible for moistening and lubricating the system. It helps digestion and keeps the body clean and pure. Mucus is especially found around the vascular system in the head, neck, and respiratory system. Mucus provides an alternative route for the return of tissue-fluid to the bloodstream. To some degree, it shares in the functioning of the circulatory system and helps to regulate body temperature. Mucus distributes hormones from the endocrine glands to the cells of the body. It also aids the blood in the production and transformation of antibodies.

There are five subcategories of Mucus, or Kapha, which are all supplied by the main center in the stomach.

Kledaka Kapha is found in the stomach; it helps in the conversion of food into a pulpy material. With the aid of Kledaka Kapha, the stomach is able to churn the food. Kledaka Kapha completes the digestion of food and is consumed in the upper digestive tract and in the small intestine.

Avalambaka Kapha is located in the heart, chest, and lower back regions that filter out the nutrients from the blood's chemical soup to provide energy to the heart. It is also found in the head and in the joints. Avalambaka Mucus helps to balance the body temperature. It also helps in the growth of bone marrow, which in turn produces disease-fighting white corpuscles that ultimately mix into the bloodstream. By a chemical reaction, this Mucus is reduced to a saline fluid and helps the blood maintain its alkaline property. Avalambaka Kapha keeps the activity level of the body high.

Bodhaka Kapha is located in the mouth, tongue, and throat, the areas that experience taste (*rasa* in Sanskrit). As saliva, this Bodhaka Kapha stimulates taste and, right from the start of the digestive process, lends softening digestive juices to food. Bodhaka Kapha takes the potent nutrients, which were isolated by Avalambaka Kapha, and alters them to provide a new, more powerful chemical to the bloodstream for distribution throughout the system. Bodhaka Kapha also works with hormones produced by the thyroid and introduces them into the blood via the vascular system.

Tarpaka Kapha is located in the head and is known as cerebrospinal fluid. *Tarpaka* in Sanskrit means "love," or "life." Tarpaka Kapha is vital life-fluid. This fluid keeps the delicate tissues of the head moist and lubricated and prevents dryness and dehydration caused by the flow of air through the nostrils. The primary function of Tarpaka Kapha is the transportation of oxygen, nutritive material, and water to the cells and of carbon dioxide and waste products to the organs of excretion. It carries positive and negative ions crucial for the proper functioning of sense organs as well. Tarpaka Kapha provides nourishment to the eyes and ears, and to the pineal, pituitary, and hypothalamus glands.

Sleshaka Kapha refers to the lubricating fluid found in the joints that saves them from wear and tear. This type of Mucus also affects the nervous system, providing power to the nerves and enabling them to receive and transmit signals. Sleshaka Kapha helps the growth of antibodies and prevents the excessive buildup of heat generated by joint activity. By means of its adhesive quality, Sleshaka Kapha serves to make the joints firm and stable.

THE SIX TASTES

A well-known Ayurvedic text states:

Poorve madhuramshniyat nadye amla lavano rasa
Ante sheshan rasan vaidyo bhojneshva char yet

During a meal, sweet tastes should be taken at the beginning, sour-tasting and salty foods should be eaten in the middle, and all the other foods—those with pungent, bitter, and astringent tastes—should be taken at the end. This is the correct order for eating foods with different tastes.

Charaka Samhita
Chapter 26, v. 43–44

All foods that we eat have a chemical nature. Although these foods contain many different chemicals, they produce only six different tastes: Sweet, Sour, Salty, Bitter, Pungent, Astringent. Each of these tastes is a combination of two of the five elements: Earth, Water, Fire, Air, and Akasha.

The Ayurvedic seers consider the subtle phenomena underlying each nutrient according to its *Rasa* (taste), *Virya* (power), and *Vipaka* (post-digestive action).* In addition to the six tastes, which refer to the effect a food has on the system *before* digestion, one of two Virya are experienced once the food enters the stomach. This refers to the sen-

---

*According to Charaka, Vipaka refers to the effect a food has on the system *after* digestion; its postdigestive effect: Sweet, Pungent, and Sour. According to Sushruta, Vipaka refers to categorizations of light (*laghu*) or heavy (*guru*).

sation of *Ushna* (hot) or *Shita* (cold). Ushna Virya has the properties of combustion, digestion, vomiting, purging; it imparts a feeling of lightness to the body and destroys semen. Ushna Virya subdues Vata (Wind) and Kapha (Mucus) and increases Pitta (Bile). Shita Virya creates steadiness and nourishment, imparts strength, increases heaviness, and aids in the buildup of body fluids. It subdues Pitta (Bile) and increases Vata (Wind) and Kapha (Mucus).

Generally, foods that have a hot taste have a Hot Virya but there are exceptions. For example, the Virya of honey is Hot, although most sweet foods have Cold Virya; the Virya of lemon is Cold, although most sour foods have a Hot Virya. The chart on page 12 shows the relationship of Tastes to Virya.

Foods are also categorized according to whether they are Dry (*shushk*) or Unctuous (*isnigdh*), and Light (*laghu*) or Heavy (*guru*).* Dry foods are mostly hot (Ushna Virya) and increase Pitta (Bile). Unctuous foods are mostly cold (Shita Virya) and increase Vata (Wind) and Kapha (Mucus). However, there are some dry foods that are cold and some unctuous foods that are hot. Light foods cause constipation, promote gas, and subdue Kapha (Mucus). Heavy foods, which subdue Vata (Wind) and Pitta (Bile), and increase Kapha (Mucus), aid in clearing urine and feces from the system. Sour-, bitter, and pungent-tasting foods are Light; salty, sweet, and astringent are Heavy. When foods are used properly, their effect can be felt on one's own system.

Sweet
Heavy, Cold, and Unctuous

The sweet taste results from the combination of water and earth. This taste is *sattvic* in nature—nourishing, soothing, and satisfying. The sweet taste provides calories, removes nervousness created by glucose deficiency, removes acidity, and provides a healthy, radiant glow to the skin. Honey and raw sugar are the best examples of this taste.

The sweet taste is congenial with the body. It increases the seven dhatus: the nutrient fluids of the body—the blood and semen—as well as the flesh, fat, bone, bone marrow, and vital essence or

ojas. It prolongs life, clarifies the sense organs, imparts vigor, and helps the complexion. It alleviates toxicosis, allays thirst and burning sensations, and helps subdue excess Vata (Wind) and Pitta (Bile).

Sweet-tasting foods have a beneficial effect on the skin, hair, voice, and strength.

Sweet-tasting foods are not good for the teeth if taken in excess. Sweet is a taste that increases Kapha (Mucus); in excess, it produces softness, lethargy, heaviness, loss of appetite, indigestion, weak gastric fire, coughs, constipation, vomiting, worms, and other diseases.

Sour
Light, Hot, and Unctuous

The sour taste results from the mixture of earth and fire. This taste is *rajasic* in nature; it excites the mind, increases appetite, produces saliva (even when a sour food is simply remembered), and helps digestion. Lemon and yogurt are the best examples of this taste.

The sour taste stimulates the digestive fire, builds up and invigorates the body, stabilizes sense functions, lightens the mind, increases strength, and regulates the movement of gases. It gives strength to the heart, encourages the production of saliva, and conducts the food downward; it moistens, digests, and gives pleasure.

If used to excess, the sour taste provokes thirst. It increases Pitta (Bile) and Kapha (Mucus) and subdues Vata (Wind). Excessive use of sour food by men is not advised because it thins seminal fluid. An excess also creates acidity in the blood and causes a general sensation of burning in the throat, chest, and heart.

Salty
Heavy, Hot, and Moist

A salty taste is produced from the merging of water and fire. This taste is rajasic and excites hunger. It attracts water and improves radiance of the skin. Rock salt, sea salt, and lake salt are the best examples of this taste.

The salty taste is a digestive; it diffuses food particles, liquefies food, and subdues Vata (Wind). It cures stiffness and obstruction of body fluids, and prevents the accumulation of toxins. It increases the secretion of saliva, liquefies mucus secretions, clarifies the digestive passage, and soft-

---

*See preceding footnote on page 9.

ens all the limbs of the body. It can easily dominate all other tastes.

If salt is used exclusively or in excess, it provokes dryness and thirst, causes fainting and body heat, increases and breaks open the skin of swellings, dislodges teeth, creates impurities of the blood, destroys virility, and impairs the functions of the sense organs. It also induces premature wrinkles, gray hair, and baldness. It is harmful for the skin and eyes, and it aggravates Pitta and Kapha.

Pungent
Light, Hot, and Dry

The pungent taste is a combination of air and fire. This taste is *rajasic-tamasic* in nature and excites the sense organs. When taken in pure form, one bite is enough to make the eyes water and the nose run. Pungent foods increase circulation and make one sweat. They dry up wounds and kill worms in the upper and lower digestive tracts. Black peppercorns, ginger, and red chilis are the best examples of this taste.

The pungent taste purifies the mouth, stimulates the gastric fire, promotes desiccation of food, and sharpens the sense organs. It gives relish to food, removes intestinal obstructions, helps elimination, and subdues Kapha (Mucus).

If used in excess, pungent foods cause a burning sensation and thirst in the throat, a dryness of mouth and lips, intense body heat, and gastritis. They are harmful for the eyes and seminal fluid; because of their postdigestive effect, an excess of pungent foods can destroy virility. An excess of this taste creates Vata (Wind) and Bile (Pitta) disorders.

Bitter
Light, Cold, and Dry

The bitter taste is produced from a blend of air and akasha (ether). This taste is rajasic in nature and excites the nervous system. As a blood purifier, it rids the body of toxins and destroys intestinal worms. Bitter foods cure diseases caused by excess Pitta (Bile) and Kapha (Mucus). Coffee and quinine are good examples of this taste.

Although the bitter taste is not pleasant, it is appetizing in its action. It is an antidote to poison and vermicide; it cures burning, itching, dermatosis, and thirst. It gives firmness to the skin and flesh. It is a digestive, a stimulant, and purifies milk in the breasts of the mother.

If used to excess, the bitter taste has a drying effect on the body; it induces weariness, fainting, and giddiness. It dries the mouth and creates Vata (Wind) disorders, which result in nervousness and loss of strength.

Astringent
Heavy, Cold, and Dry

The astringent taste is produced from a mixture of air and earth. This taste is rajasic in nature and excites the vascular system. It purifies the blood, helps the skin, and aids digestion and the assimilation of fats and oils. Alum, unripe bananas, and pomegranates are good examples of this taste.

The astringent taste is a sedative for the blood; it decreases Pitta (Bile) and Kapha (Mucus), and consumes fluids.

In excess, the astringent taste afflicts the heart, distends the stomach, impairs virility, and causes retardation of metabolic functions; it engenders various Vata (Wind) disorders. If overused, astringent foods cause dryness of mouth, palate, and lips. They cause constipation and thirst and create a change in body color.

Thus we see that the six tastes are directly responsible for the operation of and balance among the three doshas: Vata, Pitta, and Kapha.

Vata (Wind) is stimulated by astringent, bitter, and pungent tastes and subdued by sweet, sour, and salty tastes.

Pitta (Bile) is stimulated by pungent, sour, and salty tastes and subdued by sweet, astringent, and bitter tastes.

Kapha (Mucus) is stimulated by sweet, sour, and salty tastes and subdued by bitter, pungent, and astringent tastes.

These six tastes can be beneficial if they are administered in proper dosages; otherwise, they can be injurious. An intelligent and creative cook will provide all six tastes in foods rather than sticking to only a few—say, just sweet, salty, and sour tastes. Unless we use all tastes in turn, some taste buds will remain unsatisfied and the system will certainly experience a chemical deficiency. A balanced meal should include all tastes—some in large quantities, some in smaller, according to their potencies. Foods with one taste should not be used exclusively, except when fasting.

Composition, Qualities, and Effects of the Six Tastes

Attributes

- **Hot foods** cause heat in the body, excite Bile, and cure cold. These foods are suitable for mucus-dominated individuals (Kaphas).
- **Cold foods** cause cold in the body, excite Mucus, and cure heat. These foods are suitable for bile-dominated individuals (Pittas).
- **Hot and unctuous foods** are soothing, oily, and calming and cure diseases of Wind and pains of all kinds. These foods are suitable for the wind-dominated individual (Vata).
- **Cold and unctuous foods** are cooling and viscous and cure heat and dryness. They aggravate Mucus and are suitable for the bile-dominated individual (Pitta).
- **Hot and dry foods** are drying and dehydrating and cure diseases caused by mucus. These foods are suitable for the mucus-dominated individual (Kapha).
- **Cold and dry foods** are drying and cooling. These foods aggravate Wind and pain and are suitable for the bile- and mucus-dominated individual (Pitta and Kapha).

Taste	Elements	Attributes (Gunas)	Essence (Virya)	Effect (Vipak)	Vata	Pitta	Kapha	Mode of Energy (Guna)
Sweet	Earth and Water	Heavy, Cold Unctuous	Cold	Sweet Heavy	Subdues	Subdues	Increases	Sattvic
Sour	Earth and Fire	Light, Hot Unctuous	Hot	Sour Light	Subdues	Increases	Increases	Rajasic
Salty	Water and Fire	Heavy, Hot Unctuous	Hot	Sweet Heavy	Subdues	Increases	Increases	Rajasic
Pungent	Air and Fire	Light, Hot Dry	Hot	Pungent Light	Increases	Increases	Subdues	Rajasic Tamasic
Bitter	Air and Akash	Light, Cold Dry	Cold	Pungent Light	Increases	Subdues	Subdues	Rajasic
Astringent	Air and Earth	Light, Cold Dry	Cold	Pungent Light	Increases	Subdues	Subdues	Rajasic

FOODS & SPICES ACCORDING TO THEIR ATTRIBUTES

Hot and Unctuous (Subdues Vata)	Almonds,* Apples, Beets, Black cumin, Coconut (dried), Eggs, Figs, Fish, Ghee, Honeydew melon, Kidney beans, Malai (scum of cooked milk), Mango, Meat, Milk (buffalo and goat), Peanuts, Pine nuts, Pistachios, Rock sugar candy, Sago, Sesame seeds, Sweet potatoes, Urad beans (whole and split, unpeeled), Wheat
Cold and Unctuous (Subdues Pitta)	Bitter melon (karela), Butter, Buttermilk, Coconut (fresh), Cucumber, Grapefruit (sweet), Flaxseeds, Ice cream, Lemons, Locast, Lychee, Oranges, Panir (milk cheese), Peaches, Pomegranate (sweet), Pumpkin, Radishes, Spinach, Squash, Tinda (round summer squash), Water (fresh), Watermelon, Zucchini
Hot and Dry (Subdues Kapha)	Anise, Alcohol, Black pepper, Cinnamon, Dates (dried), Eggplant, Fenugreek, Ginger powder, Gram (chick-peas and chick-pea flour), Grapes, Grapefruit (sour), Honey, Kohlrabi, Lentils, Mint, Mustard greens, Onions, Peas (dried), Pickles (all types), Red pepper, Salt, Tea, Walnuts
Cold and Dry (Subdues Pitta and Kapha)	Barley, Berries, Cauliflower, Coriander, Corn, Ice, Lotus roots, Pears, Pomegranate (sour), Rosewater, Tamarind, Vinegar
Neutral	Cow's milk, Moong (mung) beans, Tomatoes, Turnips

---

*When almonds (soaked and peeled) and jaggery (raw cane sugar) are made into a cold drink, they become cold in nature and remove heat and dryness from the body.

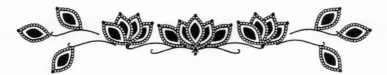

Chapter Two

BALANCED NUTRITION

While medicines help the organism fight decay and disease, the job of remaining healthy is carried out by the organism itself. The human body is self-sufficient, autonomous, and auto-synchronous in nature. Our systems are constructed in such a way that if we get enough nutrients for our tissues and fibers, if our blood circulates well, if our breathing is correct, and if we expel our toxins and waste materials properly and regularly, we should be able to enjoy a full life span—about 100 years.

Most diseases are the result of wrong eating habits and/or of eating antagonistic foods. By changing our food habits and understanding the qualities of foods and how they interact with each other, we can, up to a certain age, cure the human organism without medicines. If properly cooked food is taken in season and in the right quantities, the likelihood of falling ill is minimal.

A well-known Ayurvedic text, the *Sushruta Samhita*, states:

> By changing dietary habits the human organism may be cured without using any medicine, while with hundreds of good medicines diseases of the human organism cannot be cured if the food is wrong. Right food is the only key to good health.

According to the scholarly authors of the classic Ayurvedic texts—Sushruta, Charaka, and Vagbhatta—ingesting the proper amount of food is the key for good health. There should be a correct balance of nutrients for the seven constituent parts of the body, or dhatus: Plasma, Blood, Flesh, Fat, Bone, Marrow, and Semen.

We need foods that yield energy, that fuel our systems, that provide us with proteins, fats, and carbohydrates. To build up the body, repair the worn-out parts, and regulate the bodily processes, we need proteins, minerals, water, and cellulose.

PROTEINS

During digestion, proteins are broken down into chemical compounds called amino acids. Amino acids are molecules that make up the building blocks of protein. Body tissues cannot be built without them. Those amino acids that cannot be produced within the body must be supplied by food. These are called the eight essential amino acids. Foods that contain all of these essential amino acids are called complete protein foods. Those that lack one or more of the essential amino acids are incomplete protein foods.

Complete proteins help in building up the body. The need for complete proteins is greatest from prenatal life through childhood, when there is much new growth of bones, muscles, skin, and hair. Incomplete proteins do not contain all the essential amino acids in the correct proportions; hence, they do not efficiently repair worn-out or torn tissues and fibers. However, whatever one food lacks another can provide. By carefully combining different complementary foods, our nutritional intake can be complete.

Proteins are not stored in the body as proteins, they are stored as fats. These fats are broken down by the digestive system into amino acids only when needed. Each protein has its own pattern of amino acids: Brain protein differs from muscle protein, and muscle protein differs from blood protein. These differences reflect different combinations of amino acids.

Starting with the amino acids taken into the bloodstream, the body builds up specific proteins for different purposes. There are about eighteen different amino acids found in dietary proteins, varying in proportion and type, as well as in the order in which they are arranged.

Protein needs are greatest for women during pregnancy and lactation. These needs may be satisfied easily by a judicious combination of protein-providing foods.

Ayurvedic texts state that proteins are needed in quantity by the human body until thirty-five years of age. Using large amounts of protein after this age is useless and harmful; after thirty-five, or forty, one should use the following sources of protein:

Grains: Amaranth, Barley, Gram, Wheat

Beans: Garbanzo, Lentils, Moong (mung), Soybeans, Split peas, Sweet peas, and all Beans (fresh or dried).

The protein content in fresh beans is high and easily digestible.

Sources of Complete Protein (Lacto-Vegetarian)

Brewer's Yeast (also yeast flakes)
Butter
Buttermilk
Cheese
Cream
Ghee
Gram
Milk
Nuts (certain kinds)
Soybeans (cooked)
Soybean flour
Wheat germ
Yogurt

Protein Foods

Vegetables: Carrots, Greens (all kinds), Potatoes, Red Beets, Turnips

Nuts and seeds: Almonds, Cashews, Peanuts, Pine Nuts, Pistachios, Pumpkin, Sesame, Sunflower, Walnuts

According to information from the U.S. Department of Food and Agriculture, meat, milk, and fish contain all eight essential amino acids and all vegetables contain some of them. By consuming a variety of fresh vegetables and legumes, we can derive the important benefits of these essential amino acids. Soybeans have a higher protein content than meat.

CARBOHYDRATES

The role of carbohydrates in the body is to provide energy; they also play a small role in the growth of the body. Carbohydrates are the starches and sugars that provide the body with its most readily digestible fuel. Foods rich in carbohydrates must be chewed for a long time to assimilate the digestive juices from the saliva, thus helping the digestive process. A high-carbohydrate diet will eventually produce fat. The process of converting carbohydrates into fat occurs mainly in the liver. Muscles also store glucose as glycogen. When carbohydrates are present in excessive amounts, a diet becomes imbalanced.

Fiber

Apart from easily digestible carbohydrates, some foods contain a type of carbohydrate called fiber, which consists mostly of cellulose—the indigestible, insoluble framework of plants. This substance encourages the contraction and relaxation of the intestines, forcing the waste content of the stomach through the system. Leafy vegetables, fruits, condiments, and spices are rich in roughage. There is comparatively less roughage in cereals, root vegetables, and nuts and oily seeds, such as mustard and sesame.

Sugars

Sugars are classified as either Glucose, Fructose, Sucrose, Maltose, or Lactose. These sugars are necessary to provide the system with energy.

Glucose, a simple sugar, is carried by the blood to wherever there is activity. Glucose is found in raisins and sweet grapes. All sugars are converted into glucose before they are used in the body tissues.

Fructose is found in honey, fruits, and certain plants and vegetables. Fructose is easily assimilated and may be absorbed through the stomach walls and in the digestive tract.

Sucrose is found in sugar cane, maple sugar, and red beets.

Maltose is found in all sprouted grains. Maltose is created in all grains during the process of sprouting and starch digestion.

Lactose is found only in milk. Less quickly digested than plant carbohydrates, lactose also produces more fat.

Sugar should be used in small quantities by those who do little physical work or exercise. Jaggery (gur), or raw cane sugar, is lumpy and has a slight molasses taste; sucanot refers to organic, evaporated sugarcane juice.

If there is an excess of sugar provided by the diet, it can be stored as glycogen, or it can help form fat.

Starches

Rich sources of starch are wheat, rice (and other grains), beans, potatoes, sweet potatoes, artichokes, and dried fruits.

Several starchy foods should not be eaten together; one kind of starch, combined with dal, vegetables, and spices, makes for a balanced meal. If the diet contains a lot of carbohydrates, less butter, ghee, or oils should be used, and vice versa.

FATS

Fats are found in oils, vegetables, grains, nuts, and seeds, as well as in butter, ghee, cream, and certain tropical fruits. Fats are an excellent means of storing energy. For increasing weight, fats are better than carbohydrates because they are a concentrated source of energy. Carbohydrates can be converted into fats in the body, as anyone with a diet rich in carbohydrates discovers sooner or later.

Fats provide heat and maintain the body temperature. They provide calories and save the protein from being used as fuel. Fats convert carotene (provitamin A) in the body to vitamin A and provide the system with vitamins D, E, and K. A layer of fat under the skin provides heat insulation. Fats also save the body from dryness and dehydration and provide a protective padding around the vital organs.

The five kinds of fats, listed according to highest food value, are: butter, ghee, natural oils, hydrogenated oils, animal fat. Of these, butter, when very fresh and in its raw form, is the best. The fat content of this type of butter is easily digestible, except when used in cooking. Next comes ghee, which is harder to digest than butter but better for cooking and more easily digestible than vegetable oils. It can also be stored for a long time without refrigeration. Among vegetable oils, almond oil is superior in digestibility, followed by sesame, peanut, and mustard. After these natural vegetable oils come hydrogenated oils.

Animal fats are the most difficult fats to digest. They tax the system by needing more heat to break down and soften. When coming in contact with body temperature, lard, for instance, remains hard, while the other fats become soft.

For a healthy individual, moderate consumption of ghee or butter is not harmful. If easily digested, they make the body strong and provide vitality. But if the system is not able to digest these fats properly, then their use becomes harmful; they can damage the digestive system and create liquid stools, dysentery, weak teeth, and diabetes.

Fats are needed in the quantity of 1½ to 2 ounces per day. It is possible for people who eat a combination of dried fruits, nuts, and seeds to obtain from these foods enough fat for their needs. People who eat wheat and yogurt, or take buttermilk and other dairy products, also get enough fat. Those who are fond of ghee and butter should do work, exercise, or play games that require expenditure of physical energy.

People who do not do strenuous physical exercise do not need ghee or butter (unless they spend long hours in mental work, taxing their brain power); they may eat raisins, dried fruits, and nuts and seeds (soaked in water, then finely ground). These foods must be consumed in small quantities, or in a quantity one is able to digest.

For those who work with their brains, ghee and butter are a necessity. However, intake should not exceed one-third to one-half cup daily, depending on one's weight and digestive ability.

Too much animal fat in the diet can raise the level of cholesterol in the blood, thus narrowing and hardening blood vessels, creating heart troubles, and increasing blood pressure. However, fats from nonhydrogenated vegetable oils contain polyunsaturated fatty acids, which do not significantly increase blood cholesterol levels, even when consumed in large quantities.

VITAMINS AND MINERALS

The way the human body functions is very complex. For energy, we need food. Once food has been properly digested the nutrients are absorbed as juices and converted into blood by the liver. The blood is circulated throughout the body giving it all the energy it needs to function.

Vitamins are provided naturally in the foods we eat. Although we find no mention of vitamins in Ayurvedic texts, the way ancient peoples combined legumes, rice, wheat, butter, oil, vegetables, fruits, nuts, seeds, and spices created a fully balanced diet, complete with the vitamins required according to our modern standards. In today's world we tend toward whatever method is most expedient—usually that means we swallow a handful of factory-made pills. A better alternative is to seek a balance in diet through eating uncontaminated, organically grown foods. Research on the use of synthetic vitamins and supplements shows that they can cause harm to the system. Alarmingly, there are indications that artificial nutrients may actually contribute to the growth and development of cancer cells.

Vitamins are organic compounds found in minute quantities in fresh foods. While the body needs them only in minute quantities, vitamins function as important links in several body processes that are necessary for the health and well-being of the organism. Vitamins are either water-soluble or fat-soluble. The vitamin B complex and vitamin C belong to the water-soluble group; vitamins A, D, E, and K belong to the fat-soluble group. Most good nutrition books contain lists of foods that are high in each of these vitamins.

Minerals help the body grow and develop and also help in regulating the body processes. Minerals work through the body's enzyme system and are mostly taken in the form of salts. In vegetables and plants they exist as salts, and the body can assimilate them only in this form. The primary minerals are calcium, phosphorus, iron, iodine, sodium, potassium, sulfur, and magnesium.

WATER

Water makes up 68 percent (some authorities say 81 percent) of the total weight of the human body. The earth is composed of three parts water to one part land; the ratio in the human body is roughly the same.

The Sanskrit term for water is *jeevan*. Jeevan also means "life," so water is life. In the *Atharva Veda* it is written:

> Water is medicine, it cures diseases.
> It is also a destroyer,
> so let water free you from
> the clutches of dangerous diseases.

When the total annihilation of Creation occurs, all the earth will be submerged in water. In the beginning, too, after the ball of fire had cooled off, there was water—only water. Earth emerged much later. Since life originated in water, it is rightly called jeevan.

According to Ayurveda, water is heavy. When we pour oil on water, the oil floats; even heavy pieces of wood float on water. Water is soft, flowing, cold; it is also a good general solvent, dissolving most chemicals. All the chemical reactions of the body take place in a water-based solution. Waste products are removed from the body by water in the form of urine and sweat. Water is present in all foods, as it is a binding material. Water can be rich in minerals if obtained from a spring, well, river, or sweet water lake.

Water cleanses the system and provides nourishment. With the support of minerals, water aids in the building and repair of tissue.

Cold water activates the endocrine glands. A cold water bath cools the blood in the peripheral capillaries. This cooled blood reaches the carotid artery, which supplies the brain.

A drop in temperature activates the hypothalamus, which receives messages from the thermosensitive area of the brain. The nerve message travels to the medullae of the adrenal glands, stimulating the release of adrenaline. In turn, this causes a constriction in the peripheral blood vessels, preventing heat loss, and stimulates the kidneys to produce more urine (urinating before taking a cold bath is, therefore, advised). The kidneys also concentrate the blood by making more oxygen available to the tissues. Simultaneously, the whole endocrine system becomes activated. The pituitary gland is stimulated to produce thyrotropin, which, in turn, stimulates the thyroid. Thus a cold-water bath is a good way to activate the body.

Before meditation, a bath in water at room temperature, or slightly below room temperature (cool), is recommended. Bathing in rivers creates even higher vibrations.

Warm water cleanses the stomach and is recommended for people of cold temperament (Vatas) and mucous-dominated people (Kaphas). Warm water baths are recommended for older people anytime and for anyone during the cold weather. Taking a bath in lukewarm water was highly favored within the ancient Greek system of medicine. Since baths in lukewarm water increase virility and sexual power, they are not recommended for those wishing to meditate. Warm baths tend to weaken the nervous system, promote premature aging, and weaken digestion (unless rose water is added to the bath).

In hot climates, one should drink at least ten cups of water each day. For all other climates, six cups will suffice.

Drinking water slowly, with enjoyment and appreciation, increases the life force; it makes a medicine out of water. Water is used as a part of all healing systems. Naturopaths use it freely, as it helps the body to expel toxins.

One should not drink water:

Just after waking up
Immediately after exercise
Following an attack of diarrhea
Within 25 minutes of taking an enema
Immediately before or after urinating
After sexual intercourse .
Half-an-hour before or after meals
After hot drinks
After taking milk, cream, butter, dried
    fruits, fruits, or sweets
After eating a cucumber, honeydew, or
    cantaloupe

Those who drink too little water suffer from constipation. Those who wish to remain healthy should drink water at least an hour after both the morning and evening meals.

SALT

Salt plays a great role in the growth and development of the human body, especially in bone growth. Flesh and blood have a salty taste. The growth of the tissues that make fibers, muscles, and cells is dependent upon salt. Salt is as necessary to our cells as water. Salt helps maintain the water content of the body, which keeps us alive. If one's salt intake becomes too low, disease is sure to take over. Salt helps maintain the right amount of nutrients in the body. In all the foods we eat, salt is present in some form or other. Only in fat, oil, butter, and ghee is salt absent.

All vegetables and beans contain salt. Salt is also found in small quantities in rice. Even sugarcane (from which sugar is made) has salt in it.

For physical strength, stamina, and to gain weight, salt is necessary. This is one reason why salt is added to food. However, since salt is already present in most foods, it is not necessary to use more than one-half teaspoon of table salt per day, unless medically advised to the contrary. Sea salt, lake salt, and rock salt are commonly used in food. Of these, rock salt is reputedly the most beneficial to the human organism.

Used in proper quantities, salt increases the appetite and facilitates digestion. It also helps provide nutrients to the body, especially for vegetarians who use mostly rice, raw sugar, ghee, butter, beans, and vegetables. With the help of salt, digestive juices get converted into blood, flesh, and fat. When one is deprived of essential salt, symptoms of madness or mental disorder surface.

The intake of salt in hot weather is necessary because it is depleted through the pores of the skin as sweat. For those whose work makes them perspire, salt is necessary.

Salt has been used medically throughout the ages. Even today, saline water injections are given to terminal patients. It has been medically proven that injections of salt have helped lean people gain weight. Except for cases where certain diseases are aggravated by the use of salt, it can be used regularly by everyone.

Apart from ingesting the amounts already present in vegetables, fruits, and grains, salt should be avoided by those suffering from:

Anemia	Eye and heart
Arthritis	diseases
Coughs and colds	High blood pressure
Eczema and	Hysteria
other skin diseases	Madness
Epilepsy	Pleurisy

Salt should not be given to a person who is unconscious or in a coma. If a patient is suffering from stomach troubles, constipation, or indigestion, small amounts of salt should be used in combination with spices to energize the digestive system. When one loses more fluids than normal—by sweating, by using diuretics (foods, spices, or medicines), by loose bowels, or by vomiting—more salt can be taken daily with foods.

Salt helps protein digestion and keeps the stomach and intestines free from toxins and gases. Salt kills poisons, nourishes cells, and facilitates the growth and development of tissues. The use of salt is a must for vegetarians.

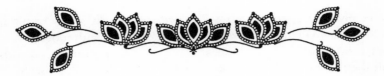

Chapter Three

FOODS AND THEIR HEALING PROPERTIES

MILK

Sweet; Cooling; Increases Mucus

According to Charaka, the great Indian sage of the Ayurvedic tradition, milk is sweet in taste and cool, light, unctuous, moderately thick, sattvic, binding, heavy (when boiled for a long period of time), and pleasant.

Milk is nectar for the human organism. Since ancient times in India, people have worshiped the cow as the Holy Mother. Protecting the cow at all costs is the highest virtue, according to Hindu religion. The cow is a divine animal that converts vegetables and plants into nutritious milk. This is why the cow is considered holy and is worshiped by Hindus. Ancient Indian medicine men placed great emphasis on milk as a healer.

The cow symbolizes Mother Earth. In many Puranic stories, whenever an imbalance between good and evil has occurred, Earth, in the form of a cow, has appeared before Lord Vishnu, the Preserver of the Universe, and asked His help in creating right balance.

In Hindu mythology, Vishnu is often depicted peacefully reclining on a serpent coiled in the Ocean of Milk. In this scene, milk symbolizes the sustaining and preserving power of the Universe. Milk is the preserver of the body.

Many of the ancient Indian sages, who compiled great works of philosophy and art, enjoyed long lives, free from anxieties and complexities. Because they worshiped and served the cow, they were rewarded by its milk, which kept them healthy and happy. Traditionally, milk has been used in India as a complete food for infants to six months of age, as well as for yogis, ascetics, and aspirants on the spiritual path.

Milk can be converted into cheese, yogurt, butter, and buttermilk; these products make up a large percentage of the foods called sattvic. Sweet dishes made from milk, such as *kheer*, constitute a good part of the diet of healthy people. In India, even now, three-quarters of the sweets sold in sweet shops are made from various combinations of milk. Milk contains plenty of calcium, protein, and vitamins; because of this combination, it is considered to be a food, a medicine, and a healer all at the same time.

Classified as one of the best elixirs, milk provides energy as soon as it goes down the throat. Not only does it provide all the ingredients needed for the growth and development of the human organism, it provides the vital life force, or ojas, and bestows longevity.

Milk is a preserver for animals as well as for human beings. All mammals, whether herbivorous or carnivorous, have milk as their first food. Even reptiles and amphibians, when they become extremely sick and cannot digest other foods, are given milk.

For children whose growth is prematurely arrested, milk is a tonic, a medicine, and a food. Indian wrestlers know the secret of milk: that it does not make people bulky and heavy, but gives them strength and increases stamina. A body built on milk has a natural shine, a glow; such a body is free from all diseases.

From the beginning of time, people have been searching for ways to live in good health and to prolong life. Yogurt, a milk derivative, has long been the secret of the Hunza. These people, who live in an isolated Himalayan kingdom and are famous for their longevity, are known to enjoy sexually active lives at the age of eighty.

Milk is a food that is readily converted into semen. It easily produces new blood, which quickens the healing processes of the body. The beauty of milk is that it affects the psyche and physique equally: It provides inner and outer strength and mental and physical power. It increases eyesight, helps growth and development, and rejuvenates the human organism.

Intolerance to Milk

Some people have difficulty digesting milk. This is because they have insufficient friendly flora in the intestine, an essential ingredient to the proper metabolic functioning of the system, or insufficient enzymes. This might be the reason there are so many diverse cultural attitudes toward milk. Ayurveda clearly prohibits the use of milk after taking nonvegetarian food, especially after seafood.

For those who cannot consume milk or dairy products, it is alright to avoid them. For those who can use milk, but suffer from problems related to mucus, it is good to use homemade cottage cheese and whey. Milk taken with a pinch of saffron or milk in which fresh basil leaves have been boiled is somewhat more digestible.

Milk in Ayurveda

A milk fast, or milk *kalpa*, is a form of treatment used by homeopaths and Ayurvedic physicians for patients who have completely lost hope of living a healthy and happy life. Extremely weak or very elderly people should not go on a milk fast, nor should people suffering from chronic diseases, or those recovering from an operation. Otherwise, it is good to fast on milk for forty days as a means of purification.

If used regularly and exclusively for two weeks or more, milk cleanses the digestive tract, stomach, and intestines and expels waste products and toxins from the system. This cures all diseases caused by toxic buildup and provides an environment that stimulates the natural healing power from within, thus rejuvenating the entire organism.

In certain Upanishads, such as the *Shatapatha Brahmana* and the *Taittiriya Brahmana*, milk, butter, and ghee are called *tejas*, which means "illuminating."

Premature aging can be cured easily by taking milk as a main part of the diet, or by going on a Milk Kalpa until the system reorganizes itself. It also soothes minor troubles that occur as a natural part of the aging process. There are cases of octogenarians suffering from gout (pain in the joints), chronic constipation, and loss of digestive fire (loss of appetite), having been cured by using milk as the main dietary staple.

Ayurveda recommends fresh milk fasts for the following ailments:

Gases of all kinds	Gout
Acidity	Piles
Stomach ailments	Impotence
Fever	Urinary troubles
Burning sensation	Neuralgic pains
Chronic constipation	Hysteria
Coughs	Amoebic dysentery

If fresh milk directly from the cow is not available, raw milk from the health food store should be used. The addition of freshly cracked black pepper will balance the doshas and lend a certain freshness to milk.

According to the well-known Hindu scripture, the *Bhagavad Gita*, one needs sattvic foods to ensure a long life and the maintenance of one's full strength up to the last breath. Sattvic foods are foods that contain nutrients that can be readily digested: Milk comes closest to satisfying this definition. Fruit juices are also sattvic. Certain *sadhus* in India subsist only on fruit juices, fruits, and milk and are able to maintain good health.

As a tonic, milk can be taken with food or medicines. However, when used as a medicine—during a forty-day Milk Kalpa, for example—it should be taken alone. Because of its chemical content, milk helps metabolic functions; it contains strong natural chemical substances that preserve the body.

Nutritional Value

The protein found in milk is of much better quality than that found in meat or eggs. If milk is used regularly, it provides the body with enough protein to take care of daily wear-and-tear of tissues. Proteins found in milk contain several amino acids that are necessary for the functioning of the brain and nervous system. While nonfat dry milk does not have many of the important qualities of fresh milk, it can be taken because of its protein value and calcium content.

Milk, combined with grains or potatoes in the diet, gives vegetarians optimum proteins. These proteins are more easily digestible and less toxic than those found in meat. One quart of milk satisfies almost one-third of our daily protein requirement.

The lower the fat content of the milk, the more easily it is digested by the system. For people whose work is more mental than physical, lowfat milk is better; atheletes and people who do physical labor should take whole milk, since the fats provide their systems with energy. Vitamins A and D are present in the fat of milk and in its derivatives, butter and ghee.

Drinking two cups of milk, along with eating a balanced diet, should provide the average daily requirement of calcium; when one is fasting on milk alone, 10 cups (2½ quarts) per day are needed to satisfy the calcium requirement.

Like other electrically charged elements in the body, calcium has a profound influence on the functioning of the nervous system. It is needed for the transmission of neurological messages. Milk also contains phosphorus and iron, which are good for the blood and eyes, as well as trace minerals. A small amount of digestible silver is even present in mother's milk. The water content of milk helps in the digestion of iron, iodine, and other minerals.

Milk also serves as a neutralizing agent for poisons and toxins. Milk gives strength to the glands. The digestive juices and other nutrients found in milk aid the system in fighting tuberculosis bacilli and leprosy. Milk is a diuretic; it cleans the kidneys and urinary tract by prompting urination.

Thus, we realize that milk contains all the nutrients required by the human organism. As stated earlier, milk should be taken on its own when meant to be a medicine. If taken with other medicines and/ or food, it will serve only as a tonic and purifier.

Cow's Milk

Milk is best straight from the cow, while still warm. In India, cows are revered and carefully tended. They are brushed and washed regularly and not milked once pregnant.

In Vedic times, care of the cow was a sattvic activity: There was no need to pasteurize or homogenize milk. Now milk sold in supermarkets is ultrapasteurized, which stops the natural souring process. Some claim pasteurized milk causes osteoporosis.

The vibrational effect of an electric milking machine must be shattering for the cow—imagine the difference in quality of milk from a well cared for and revered cow, hand-milked. The qualities of fresh milk are beyond words.

Boiling milk makes it easier to digest. The longer milk is cooked ucous   mucusafter the boiling point, the more powerful it becomes and also the more difficult it is to digest (unless one is getting plenty of exercise).

Milk from a cow that has just delivered a calf is especially powerful. It should not be drunk, however, until twenty-one days after calving. If this milk is consumed earlier, it is heavy and more mucus-producing. Milk taken from the mother cow between twenty-one days and four months after delivery is tasty, pleasant, unctuous, and strength-providing. Such milk increases a person's glow (*ojas*), stimulates the intellect and intuition, and lends ready wit and presence of mind.

In Ayurveda, cows are classified according to their color and where they are found. Ayurvedic scriptures give a complete account of the qualities of human milk, as well as that of donkey, sheep, horses, goats, camels, and elephants (see Appendix C).

Curative Qualities of Milk

Whenever the organism becomes tired or depleted, regular ingestion of milk rejuvenates and allows it to become active again. One main cause of premature aging stems from deposits of food materials in the intestinal walls. This condition paralyzes the process of assimilation—the main job of the intestines. When digestion is poor, various organs are unable to receive their proper supply of nutrients and thus start aging quickly. If waste materials that stick to the intestinal walls are expelled properly, all the organs will receive a proper food supply, and the problem of premature aging will be removed or will not arise.

Milk cleanses the digestive tract. It expels toxins and waste products from the stomach and intestines and supplies the body with a nutritious material that is readily digestible and easily convertible into blood. Since milk proteins contain many amino acids and milk is alkaline in nature, it aids the stomach during digestion. In fact, it helps during all stages of digestion—in the mouth, stomach, and small intestine. And if the digestive system is working properly, the circulatory system works. If the circulatory system works, so does the nervous system. These three systems regulate the human organism, and milk, thus, indirectly regulates them all.

Diseases reach the human body by means other than the external invasion of bacteria and viruses. Accumulation of poisons and toxins, irregularity of bowel movements, improper dietary habits, negative thoughts, an unhealthy atmosphere, emotional suppression, stale or rotten food, and lack of exercise are some of the many factors that render the body susceptible to disease.

The human organism is auto-synchronous; if the body is accumulating toxins, purification is needed. Disease is a natural purification device— a warning that something in the system needs to be corrected. In addition to intestinal, kidney, urinary, gallbladder, and gynecological problems, the following afflictions can often be cured with proper use of milk:

Anemia	Nervousness
Asthma	Obesity
Colds	Paralysis
Coughs	Premature aging
Gout	Tuberculosis
Impotency	Weak digestive fire
Jaundice	Wrinkles
Liver problems	

Children's diseases caused by weak constitution, malnutrition, and ill health of the mother in pregnancy are also curable with milk fasts.

Generally, milk fasts can cure nervous diseases—insomnia, neurosis, headaches, irritability, dullness, swelling of the hands and feet, toughness of the nerves and muscles, and pessimism. These fasts are also said to cure diseases of the stomach—peptic ulcers, intestinal ulcers, and acidity. As well, milk fasts cure displacement of the womb,

chronic constipation, dysentery, potbelly, diseases of the liver, chronic amoebic dysentery, diabetes, swelling of the kidneys, lack of vitality and virility, diseases affecting the menstrual cycle, and freckles. They also cure postnatal problems found in the mother, such as waist pains, excess weight, unattractiveness, impurities in the blood, and general weakness, as well as the effects of miscarriage.

In sum, many diseases sometimes can be cured by milk fasts, even tuberculosis and cancer, providing the milk is fresh and the cow is not fed with formula foods. Diseases of the heart are the exception. They are caused by improper circulation and a blockage of blood flow through the arteries and veins; since milk does not travel through arteries and veins, it cannot clean and purify them.

Ghee
Sweet; Cooling; Increases Mucus, in excess
Ghee, or clarified butter, is the best cooking medium. It has a most delicate flavor and keeps for months or even years without refrigeration. Ghee is made from butter, but traditionally in India it is made from the butter of yogurt, not of milk.

Ghee, available at health food stores and Indian groceries, has been used for more than 6,000 years in India. It is highly praised in Ayurvedic scriptures for its purifying, disinfecting, and healing properties. For internal purposes, it is best taken when relatively fresh (up to one year old). Fresh ghee applied regularly to the eyelids with a clean fingertip is excellent for eyesight. It is also used to cure other ailments of the eyes. When ghee is over one year old, it is best used externally, such as in massage. For massage designed to treat certain diseases, ghee that is two-to -three-years old is preferred. (See page 73 for instructions on how to make ghee.)

Yogurt
Sour, astringent; Cooling;
Increases Mucus and Bile
Yogurt possesses the same food values as milk— protein, calcium, and a wealth of B vitamins. Fresh yogurt is alkaline; as it sours, it becomes more acidic and aggravates Bile (Pitta). Yogurt has a general invigorating effect on the system. It is more readily digestible than fresh milk and furnishes valuable bacteria, which aid in the assimilation of many nutrients, to the intestines.

Yogurt made at home from fresh milk provides

most of the nutrients required by the human system. It serves well as a basic item in a summer diet. Yogurt made from raw milk has the highest nutritional value and provides a lot of energy. Yogurt made at home from pasteurized milk is preferable to that found in stores, which may be old, sour, and made from skimmed and/or powdered milk products.

Yogurt can be eaten alone or can serve as a base for fruit salads or raitas. It is best served before sunset.

Yogurt increases Kapha (Mucus) and therefore is not good for people suffering from colds and coughs or those with kapha-dominated temperaments. Because its sourness stimulates Pitta, it is not recommended for people with Pitta disorders. Yogurt should always be taken with a little salt, cumin, or black pepper, or, if a sweet taste is desired, with saffron and honey or raw sugar.

GRAINS

Wheat
Sweet; Cooling; Increases Mucus

Wheat has justly been called the "monarch" of foods. No other dietary staple, except fresh yogurt and buttermilk, provides such concentrated nourishment for all seven of the body constituents, or dhatus. Of all grains and cereals, wheat is the most readily digestible by the human system because of its capacity to absorb water, which, in turn, conducts heat uniformly through the grain.

Wheat is a food that should not be eaten fresh. The grain freshly plucked from the stalk contains more solar energy than the human system can adequately process. Therefore, wheat should be eaten only after it has been aged for at least four months. If this is not possible, wheat should be soaked in water overnight, then sun-dried for three days before being converted into wheat flour and used for making breads. Since stored and water-soaked wheat remains fertile, the excessive solar energy is discharged into the atmosphere instead of the stomach. So great is the solar energy concentrated in wheat that granaries storing vast quantities of this nutritious food must be continuously ventilated; otherwise, spontaneous combustion could generate fire or even explosions in the freshly ground flour.

In whatever form wheat is taken, it should first be thoroughly browned. Breads are best toasted.

Preferably, thin, tortilla-like breads ought to be prepared fresh for each meal. These breads may be roasted dry, or in a lightly oiled pan over medium heat. Wheat cereals should be browned in a dry (unoiled) pan over medium heat before adding water. Cracked wheat prepared in this fashion provides an excellent breakfast food.

Wheat is sweet in taste, cooling in effect, and heavy. It is rich in vitamins, minerals, proteins, carbohydrates, and many other nutrients. It can be taken with any meal on any occasion. The gluten content in wheat provides the body with physical endurance and sexual stamina. For this reason, celibates should eat smaller amounts of wheat products than married individuals, unless they are engaged in hard physical labor. Persons wishing to reduce their gluten intake should use coarsely ground whole wheat flour, since in this form less gluten is assimilated.

Wheat Flour
Sweet; Cooling; Increases Mucus

Wheat flour contains vitamins B and E in sufficient quantities to provide heat and energy for the body. Whenever possible, stone- or hand-ground whole wheat flour should be used. Before the dough is made, the flour needs to be sifted through a medium-mesh sieve; this procedure will allow the nutritious wheat germ to pass through, along with the flour. This sieved flour is easily digestible.

When making Indian breads, such as chapatis, the wheat dough preferably is made about two hours before cooking. This will help make the bread light and easy to digest, so that the stomach and intestines do not have to waste extra energy in breaking down and assimilating. Also, while rolling the dough, dusting flour should be used sparingly since too much of it will make the bread heavy and spoil the stomach.

If desired, 1 teaspoon of salt can be added to 2 pounds of wheat flour to make the bread tastier, easier to digest, and more energy-giving.

Wheat can be stored, but once converted into flour, it should not be kept for more than fifteen days. Packages of wheat flour sold in supermarkets should not be used, as they are sure to be over fifteen days old. Freshly ground wheat flour, obtained from a farmhouse or health food store, should be used within two weeks. One can also purchase the wheat berries (unprocessed whole wheat kernels) and grind them at home when needed.

Whole wheat flour is preferable to the enriched white varieties. Fresh, whole-grain, homemade bread is always better than store-bought bread. The finely ground white flour usually sold in supermarkets does not contain the husk of the wheat. For this reason it sticks to the walls of the stomach and intestines and is hard to digest and constipating. Most commercial breads found in hotels and restaurants are made from finely ground white flour. Avoid them. If finely ground white flour must be used for baking bread, add one teaspoon of ajwain seeds to 2½ cups of wheat flour. This will remove the constipating effect, rendering it digestible.

Rice
Sweet; Cooling; Increases Mucus

Rice, more than any other grain, is an international food. All varieties of rice are digestible, and only occasionally are they constipating. People with gastritis can tolerate rice when it is cooked with ½ cup of coconut powder and a few whole cloves for every 2 cups of uncooked rice. Rice cures and removes heat. Brown rice is regarded as healthy because the husk stays intact. Along with the luxurious wild rice (which is actually a grass), it takes a longer time to digest. Dals (beans) with skin and whole wheat flour contain the same vitamins as brown rice. Basmati, available at health food stores and Indian groceries, is a richly scented rice that is easy to digest; handpounded and unpolished white Basmati, which contains the husk, is best for cooking and is the kind intended to be used in all of the rice recipes in this book.

It is always advisable to let rice age. There is a saying: "Wood, rice, and wine improve in quality when they are old." The best rice is rice that has been stored (in its unpounded, unpolished form) for at least one to two years before being consumed. The husk is removed by hand pounding just before use.

All varieties of rice are sweet in taste, cool in action, and provide vitamins A and B. These vitamins are lost, however, in polished rice. When rice is cleaned and polished by machine its best part is removed, and the whole grain is reduced to white rice. This outer layer, called the husk, provides the very substance that saves the human body from skin diseases and gives energy to the brain. Handcleaned, unpolished rice is best. However, if dal

(any kind) with skins are combined with an equal amount of the polished rice, the required amount of A and B vitamins can be obtained, thus compensating for the loss.

When rice is cooked as *pulao* (pilaf), the peas, nuts, and seeds that are added while cooking provide the proteins and vitamins not present in rice. Of all grains, rice has the least power or energy-giving potential, but when taken with milk, nuts, and seeds, or saffron, this potential increases. Boiled rice is very good.

Made into a sweet dish, such as kheer or pudding, rice is spectacular. Because rice is cold (lunar), its use should be avoided in cold climates.

Persons anxious to lose weight can eat rice boiled without salt, sugar, or spices. In cases of chronic dysentery or tuberculosis, old rice cooked with dal in the form of *khichari* is beneficial. For diarrhea or loose bowels, rice and yogurt are ideal foods, but they are poison when taken during a fever or when suffering from a cold.

FRUITS

Apricots
Sweet, astringent; Heating; Increases Bile

Apricots are a favorite food in the northwest Himalayas. They have been used there for centuries as a staple food because they provide a great deal of nourishment. Apricots are similar in shape to peaches and also have a pit inside. The pits are sold in the market and oil is extracted from the kernel. This oil is as good as almond oil.

Fresh apricots subdue excess Vata (Wind) and Kapha (Mucus). Rich in protein, carbohydrates, sodium, calcium, magnesium, phosphorus, sulfur, copper, iron, and chlorine, they are also an excellent source of vitamin A. Dried apricots contain three times more vitamin A than fresh ones. Taken in large quantities (from six to twelve) by patients with chronic constipation, dried apricots help evacuation. (Vatas can have dried fruit if it is soaked first.) They help anemic patients because of their rich iron and calcium content, and also increase the production of hemoglobin.

For ease in chewing and assimilation, dried apricots must be soaked overnight before serving. Before soaking, they must be properly rinsed. The water in which they are soaked, rendered rich with apricot juice, can be drunk. Dried apricots are most easily digested when boiled or soaked in milk.

Soaked apricots can be used in salads and chutneys, and in place of tamarind when making *saunth*. The compressed pulp of apricots is very good for making saunth (see recipes on pages 197 and 198).

Bananas
Sweet, astringent; Cooling;
Increase Mucus and, in excess, Bile

Bananas are a holy food and are very popular in India as *prasad* (consecrated food). They are useful in cases of dysentery, diarrhea, chronic indigestion, and in general for people suffering from weak digestive fire. As a fruit they are a great tonic and provide the system with large amounts of nutrients.

Ripe bananas are popular everywhere. Size and shape differ depending on where they are grown. The ones with a golden yellow skin and brown spots are among the best tasting.

According to Ayurvedic texts, bananas are tasty, appetizing, and fibrous. They are a flesh-building fruit and quench the thirst. They are good for diseases caused by excess Wind (Vata); in excess they aggravate Bile (Pitta) and Mucus (Kapha) because the long-term effect of bananas is sour. Being sweet in taste, they increase the amount of semen, and thus, increase vitality and virility. Bananas cure all kinds of weaknesses, and they especially help cure diabetes and spermatorrhea.

Slightly constipating when taken in small quantities, bananas remove and cure constipation if used properly and regularly. One large banana, or two or three small bananas eaten one after the other, will remove constipation. Bananas solidify stools and may be given to children from the age of two months. Infants and grandparents without teeth can take bananas mashed or liquefied. Ripe bananas digest easily, providing one does not eat too few. Regular eating of bananas, oranges, and apples—depending on your constitution—keeps the system healthy. (Apples, for example, aggravate Vatas but are good for Pittas.)

For thin, bony people, bananas are an ideal food. Thin people should eat two bananas a day after food regularly for a few months. This will help them gain weight without getting fat and will help them look more beautiful. For those who urinate often, bananas are a very good remedy. In general,

they help reduce disease. Bananas help make people who have exhausted themselves by sexual overindulgence strong again.

For dry coughs and whooping cough, a drink made from bananas can work like an expectorant and help break up the cough.

Bananas are best eaten after other foods so they can aid in digestion. They contain plenty of calories, vitamins A, C, D, and E, and many mineral salts. Bananas contain 75 percent water, a number of carbohydrates, a small amount of protein, and very little fat. Bananas also contain B vitamins, and minerals such as calcium, phosphorus, iron, magnesium, copper, sulfur, and potassium.

Flour can be made from dried banana flakes (available in health food stores). Pancakes made from this flour are delicious and satisfying. Banana flour is more nutritious than any cereal flour. Ripe bananas with milk, nuts, and seeds, or bananas in muesli make a good breakfast treat. They are highly alkaline and help maintain the alkaline reserve in the body. Bananas are an ideal food for gastric ulcers, gastritis, and ulcerative colitis.

In cases of weak digestive fire, bananas can be given with tamarind and salt. One banana, thoroughly mashed, is a good remedy for dysentery in children.

Bananas help build bones and are very good for jaundice because of their iron content. They also aid acute gout and arthritis.

Eating bananas helps the heart; when there is pain in the heart, bananas blended with honey can be a lifesaver. With honey, they are an ideal sattvic food; a pinch of saffron may also be added.

Placing banana skins over an area with muscular pain or on an area of pain due to scratching prevents swelling and provides relief. If, by chance, one eats more than a reasonable number of bananas and experiences indigestion, the seeds of one black (or red) cardamom pod should be chewed slowly and swallowed to aid in digestion.

Coconut
Sweet; Cooling; Increases Mucus

The coconut is oily and smooth in nature. Coconuts subdue excess Wind (Vata) and Bile (Pitta). Being a holy food, the coconut is popular in India as prasad (blessed food). For worship it is taken with sugar candy or raisins. The coconut, with its rough bark and "beard" intact, is offered to Vishnu and

Shakti at their shrines or put into the river Ganga* as an offering. Coconut is worshiped as Vishnu and as Satya Narayan, the Lord of Truth. At the commencement of all ceremonies a coconut is broken, symbolizing the breaking of the ego, and is offered to God. Its pieces are then distributed to the people present. The coconut is sent as a token of good luck in Indian marriage arrangements. According to legend, this sattvic fruit is a gift from the gods to human beings.

Coconut is used daily as a food in many parts of the world. Rich in food value, coconut meat is especially high in calories and easy to digest. The protein found in coconuts is regarded as of particularly high quality because it contains all the amino acids necessary for the body. Coconut is a good source of B vitamins and several minerals. The oil content of coconuts makes them sought after by thin persons who wish to gain weight. When it is cold-pressed, the oil is easily digestible and consumed by the body with the same ease as other oils and fats. Coconuts, green or ripe, and coconut milk are excellent remedies for curing acidity in the stomach. The oil present in the milk and flesh neutralizes and reduces stomach acids.

The coconut is utilized in all stages of growth: Green coconut milk is a refreshing drink and good for the stomach because of its alkaline nature. The milk of green coconuts contains the full complement of B vitamins. These rich resources make it a rejuvenator. When tender and sweet, the pulp of a ripe coconut is eaten raw; since its sugar is in solution, digestion and assimilation are easy.

Dried coconut in grated, shredded, or powdered form (available at health food stores and Indian groceries) is good for the intestines because of its particular chemical content; the digestive residue serves as a brush to clean the intestines. It is useful in curing hiccups, vomiting, and overacidity. Coconut powder can be used in sweet dishes, rice, chutneys, confectionaries, and puddings; it also can be eaten raw.

Coconut oil is very good for the hair and for massage of the body. It is cooling when used on sunburned skin. Excellent for healing wounds, it also moisturizes the skin and is widely employed in cosmetics and shampoos.

---

*Ganges

Dates
Sweet; Cooling; Increase Mucus

Dates give power to the stomach and cure diseases of excess Wind (Vata). Normally dates increase Mucus but in conjunction with certain herbs, they can cure diseases of excess Mucus (Kapha). They are very useful for those suffering from dry coughs. Dates help to increase body weight. If followed by buttermilk, dates are immediately digested.

In India, dates are found in two main varieties: One is large, sweet, and tasty; the other is small and not so sweet. Dates are used as a sweetener and as candies in certain parts of India. They are rich in food value and satisfying. Dates increase semen and give strength, stamina, vitality, and virility. Those who have exhausted themselves from sexual overindulgence, or those who are always depressed or fatigued, should eat fifteen to twenty dates a day after meals for several months. Date sugar is easily digestible and high in calories. By doing this and taking at least 2 cups of milk, as well as exercising, within forty days one will feel rejuvenated, with both physical and mental strength restored.

In cases of injury involving much blood loss, dates and milk with a little ghee or cream will make the patient feel better immediately.

For those with anemia or general weakness, dates with milk and cream at breakfast are very helpful. For those who feel they are losing stamina, date milk is a tonic. Persons who do not have clear morning bowel movements should drink milk boiled with four or five dried dates (chuhara) before going to sleep at night.

Dates have vitamins A and B, a combination that gives the system the power to resist viruses and infections. Dates also contain protein and carbohydrates, as well as calcium, phosphorus, potassium, iron, and pectin, which makes them rejuvenators.

Dates can be used in many ways: as a sweet, with vegetables, as pickles, and in sour chutneys.

According to Ayurveda, dates combined with specific herbs can work to expel mucus and thus have a medicinal value for ailments of the chest region and coughs. Dates provide strength to the heart, liver, pancreas, and kidneys. They help in building up nerves in the brain and increase appetite. They are tissue-building. According to an Indian handbook dating from the Middle Ages, dates are cold and dry, good if taken in moderation for the intestines, and dangerous if taken in excess for the throat and chest. It recommends combining dates with comb honey; it also considers dates a most suitable food for seniors and debilitated persons, for those convalescing, and for children. Through regular use of dates, friendly bacteria become established in the intestines.

Dates are alkali-forming in nature. They maintain an alkaline balance in the system, are regarded as a health food, and serve to purify and strengthen the blood.

Wealthy Arabs eat dates filled with butter. The carbohydrate content of dates helps the digestion of butter. Dates are reputed to be a holy food. The date palm tree and the coconut palm, which belong to the same genus, are both holy trees.

Figs
Sweet, astringent; Cooling;
Increase Mucus

Figs, which are also a holy food, can be eaten fresh or dried. When dried, their nutritional value is doubled. When allowed to ripen on the tree, the fruits that are collected are either eaten or kept for drying. Ripe figs are palatable, sweet in taste, and cold in nature; they aid the digestive process and help rid the system of impurities in the blood. Figs subdue excess Wind (Vata) and Bile (Pitta). Fresh figs are best for Vatas; if they are not available, dried figs can be soaked in water overnight and then eaten.

Figs contain protein and minerals, such as sodium, potassium, calcium, iron, copper, magnesium, phosphorus, sulfur, and chlorine.

Figs are always recommended for chest troubles and for constipation. They are also good for chronic coughs. Fig syrup is an excellent tonic for infants, increasing appetite and improving digestion. This syrup also cures rheumatism, seminal disorders, skin troubles, stones in the kidney or bladder, enlargement of the liver, and leukorrhea.

It is advisable for women of all age groups to eat two figs per day. From the onset of menstruation until the onset of menopause, women should take three figs daily to compensate for the loss of certain elements in the body, such as iron and calcium. Because of the iron content in figs, they are prescribed to patients with anemia.

Figs promote quick recovery after prolonged illness. If taken in large quantities, they help thin people put on weight. Bodybuilders and wrestlers eat figs with nuts. Figs are also used as a laxative, and they help cure piles.

The skin of dried figs is very tough, so it is better to soak them overnight in clean water. Because of its rich mineral and sugar content, this water can then be drunk or used in cooking. The skin of (soaked) dried figs may be discarded, and the seeds and pulp should be thoroughly masticated.

Grapes
Sweet, sour, astringent; Cooling;
Increase Mucus

Grapes are one of the oldest and most delicious fruits known, principally because they are so rich in glucose and because of their alkaline-forming nature. The acids and glucose are thoroughly assimilated by the body and stimulate activity of the kidneys and bowels. Grapes subdue excess Wind (Vata) and Bile (Pitta).

The ancient Indian Ayurvedic scholar Vagbhatta considers grapes to be a laxative and diuretic. The wise master Sushruta considers them to be nutritious. He believes they provide the body with life force, which saves it from infection and deterioration. Organic grapes definitely help the intestines; they should be consumed by those suffering from weak digestion. The cellulose in grapes forms the inital pulp for stools. The skins should be thoroughly masticated, otherwise they will produce flatulence.

Grapes have also been found helpful in diseases of the skin and lungs, as well as in gout, rheumatism, arthritis, and obesity.

Apart from glucose and acid, grapes contain vitamins, some minerals, such as phosphorus and calcium, a negligible amount of fat, and very little protein.

In India grapes are eaten both fresh and dried. Fresh grapes are either eaten raw or are used in certain exotic drinks. Dried grapes are of two kinds: raisins and *munnaqua*. Raisins are small sun-dried grapes and are sweet/sour in taste. Munnaqua are raisins made from large, ripe, sweet grapes; they are sweet in taste. Munnaqua are often recommended by doctors. They are very tasty and nutritious. Their glucose is predigested and readily absorbed by the body. It enters into the bloodstream as soon as it reaches the stomach and gets converted into heat and energy very quickly. Therefore, munnaqua are given to older people and people suffering from fever, anemia, general weakness, weak digestion, constipation, dropsy, dysentery, colitis, bronchitis, cardiac disorders, and kidney trouble.

Fasting on grapes, or grapes and milk, for four to six days once a year is a good method of purification. One should consume two to four pounds of grapes per day during this period. Ripe, sweet grapes should be eaten fresh, or taken as juice.

Vinegar made from grape juice of the sour variety is also good when taken in small quantities with food.

Grapefruit
Sweet, bitter; Cooling;
Increases Bile and Mucus

This appetizing and refreshing member of the citrus family was developed from a large, sweet lemon tree that grows all over India. But the actual use of grapefruit in India is recent. They are grown only in Punjab and Uttar Pradesh.

Grapefruits prove to be a good substitute for oranges, having almost the same food value. They subdue excess Wind (Vata).

These fruits are an important source of vitamin C and bioflavonoids. They contain minerals, such as calcium, phosphorus, and potassium.

An alkali-forming food, grapefruit balances the acid reactions of different foods and relieves constipation. For these reasons the fruit is eaten fresh, with its pulp. Grapefruit encourages healthy intestines and prevents diarrhea, dysentery, and other infectious diseases of the digestive tract. Grapefruit has also been found useful in various diseases of the liver.

Grapefruit should be taken before other food, not after. If the juice is taken, the pulp should be taken with it. The seedless variety is healthier and preferable.

Fasting on grapefruit juice with pulp for three days is an excellent way to purify the stomach and intestines, because, in their postdigestive state, grapefruits produce an alkaline residue even though they are an acidic fruit.

A delicious grapefruit chutney is made by grinding together grapefruit, mint leaves, and fresh green or red peppers. Add to this mixture a pinch of salt and freshly ground or dried coconut powder. (While the coconut powder is optional, it increases food value and bulk.)

Grapefruit salad can be made with onions, tomatoes, and salad greens.

An ideal summer drink from grapefruit can be made either from the pure juice alone, or by mixing it with raw sugar or honey.

Lemon
Sour; Heating;
Increases Bile and Mucus

Lemons, which belong to the same family as grapefruit, are highly praised in Ayurveda for their qualities. Lemons are an appetizer—they stimulate digestion and assimilation. Lemons are healers—they calm the system and provide nutrients. Almost every part of a lemon is used for human consumption. Apart from providing juice, the peel of lemons is used for making pickles. The medicinal value of a fresh lemon is as high as that of a pickled lemon.

Lemons are good for subduing excess Wind (Vata). In all stomach disorders, pickled lemon is used as a home remedy. Its medicinal value is reputed to increase as it matures. Some sort of pickle is a must with food. Pickles tickle the tongue and encourage digestive juices and saliva. Pickling (see page 199) is an ideal way of preserving lemons and of increasing their medicinal value. It is good to take pickled lemon with the midday meal, but avoid it at breakfast and dinner.

Because lemons contain vitamin C and bioflavonoids, they prevent scurvy and capillary fragility. Lemons also contain B vitamins as well as minerals, such as sodium, potassium, magnesium, calcium, iron, copper, phosphorus, and sulfur.

Lemons are an important source of citric acid. Because of this, they are popular in medical and home remedies. Lemons relieve thirst, are cooling, soothe the nerves, and cure nausea. They are used for indigestion, acidity, dysentery, and diarrhea. Lemon juice is a sedative for the heart and reduces palpitations. The juice is helpful for people with high blood pressure and for the bowels and kidneys, uterus, and other parts of the body. Lemons stimulate the flow of saliva and cure loss of appetite and dyspepsia.

Lemons encourage secretion of bile and are, therefore, recommended for patients with jaundice. Because they convert into an alkaline substance during digestion, lemons counteract conditions such as acidity, rheumatism, and gout.

Lemon juice is an organic disinfectant that causes no harm to body tissues. It prevents the formation of stones in all parts of the body. Lemon juice checks colds and possesses an antipneumonia substance. Lemons cure gas and the juice is a mild laxative. Lemon juice taken with lukewarm water every morning cures constipation. Drinking the juice through a straw will prevent erosion of tooth enamel.

The use of lemons in salads and as a preserver is well known. A lesser known fact is that lemon seeds are especially useful in curing nausea brought on by aggravated bile and in curing repeated vomiting. A few fresh lemon seeds, peeled and ground into a fine paste in a mortar with a pestle and mixed with a teaspoonful of honey, can work miraculously in these situations.

Lemon juice taken in lukewarm water with a tablespoon of honey early each morning as the first drink of the day helps dieters lose weight. Lemons are also used in fasting. A one-week lemon-water fast cures all diseases of the stomach and intestines.

Finely sliced or chopped onions mixed with lemon juice, a pinch of salt, and some freshly sliced or chopped red or green pepper, is a very popular salad among Muslims and onion-eating Hindus.

Constant use of lemon juice with food or in food, or of lemon pickles keeps the body in good shape. In all preparations, however, the seeds should be removed. The seeds are to be used separately only for relief of nausea, as mentioned above.

A special lemon drink call Shikangibin is very popular on hot summer days in India. Shikangibin is made by adding fresh lemon juice to a sugar solution. Some powdered spices with a pinch of black salt are then sprinkled over the drink (see recipe on page 243).

Mangoes
Sweet, slightly sour; Heating;
Balance all doshas

Mangoes are unctuous, give energy, and are satisfying. A hybrid mango that has no fiber is heavy to digest, although it tastes better than one with fiber. Natural mangoes are smaller and juicier than hybrids but both usually are sweet and sour. The sweeter the mango, the more easily it is digested

and the more energy it provides. A sour mango should never be eaten, except in the form of *amchur* (mango powder) or as dried mango flakes.

Mangoes are good for excess Wind (Vata) and Mucus (Kapha). A ripe, sweet, juicy mango helps the body generate blood. If a glass of lukewarm milk is taken after eating a mango, it balances Bile (Pitta) and energizes the entire system—especially the intestines. During the hot season, cold water can be added to the milk to reduce the effects of the heat and give strength, vigor, and vitality to the system.

Mangoes stimulate and energize the nervous system and are weight-producing. They cure constipation, activate the kidneys, and prompt the flow of urine, which enables the system to flush out toxins. A drink made from a juicy mango that has a lot of fiber is a cure for people who suffer from too little digestive heat, chronic dysentery, or constipation.

Because their acid content increases stomach acids, mangoes should never be eaten on an empty stomach. They help one stay youthful for a long time, check premature aging, and hold back decay. By going on a Mango Kalpa, or fast—living on juicy, ripe mangoes in season followed by milk for forty to sixty days—one rejuvenates the stomach and intestines, increases digestive heat, and thus stimulates the appetite. Milk absorbs all the heat of mangoes and prevents stomach disorders; water should never be taken after eating a mango.

Mangoes soaked in a sugar syrup give energy; they remove constipation and are a tonic for the brain, stomach, lungs, and blood.

Papayas
Sweet, astringent, slightly bitter;
Cooling; Increase Bile

Papayas, when soft, sweet, and ripe, are a delicacy. They subdue excess Wind (Vata). Papayas are considered rich in vitamins, especially vitamin A.

Papayas also contain protein, B vitamins, vitamin C (which increases as the fruit ripens), and minerals, such as calcium, phosphorus, and iron. The carbohydrate in papayas contains mainly invert sugar, which is readily absorbed into the blood. As the fruit is exposed to the sun, it gets sweeter and richer in vitamins.

· Vaidyas (Ayurvedic doctors) and Hakims—

(physicians who practice Unani-Tib, the Greek system of medicine)—prescribe papaya to people suffering from liver, heart, and/or intestinal trouble. The fruit is also used as a cure for intestinal worms. Papaya encourages the appetite and helps digestion; it is a diuretic and prevents flatulence. Raw papaya can be used either in a curry or as a dried fruit. It is delicious in sweet dishes. Papaya has a soothing effect on the stomach and pancreas. It is used with meat and fish as a "softener" because it helps the digestion of these foods. Grated papaya cooked with milk converts the milk into cheese and makes a delicious dish that is easy to digest and also good for the intestines. Raw papaya is helpful for patients with liver trouble. It also makes the muscle fibers of the womb contract, thus aiding menstrual flow.

Warning: Raw papaya can induce abortion if taken by pregnant women.

Ripe papaya, served with cream, nuts, and seeds, is an excellent summertime breakfast. In winter, papayas should not be eaten after sunset. During the rainy season, papayas should be eaten less often because of their diuretic effect.

Peaches
Sweet, astringent; Cooling; Increase Mucus, in excess

Peaches are good for those who suffer from loss of appetite due to excessive heat in the system. Patients with fever feel energetic if they are given one peach every two hours during the day.

Peaches subdue excess Wind (Vata); however, eating two or three peaches a week is good for everyone.

Peaches are delicious in fruit salad with honey, nuts, and seeds, or in muesli. They can also be cooked with vegetables, in which case small pieces are added in place of tomatoes to the basic masala mixture while it is cooking.

Pineapple
Sweet, sour; Cooling; Increases Mucus, in excess

Pineapple cures both anxiety and a disturbed heart; it provides a cool feeling to the head and heart. It is sweet/sour in taste, and sweet in action. The pulp of pineapple quenches thirst and increases mucus. It is good to subdue excess Wind (Vata) and Bile (Pitta). Pineapple is an excellent aid to digestion

when taken in small quantities with a meal. It adds a refreshing quality to curries. Sweet pineapple can be cooked with, or as a substitute for, tomatoes.

Plums
Sweet, astringent; Cooling; Increase Mucus

Plums are cold and easily digestible. If eaten in small quantities, plums help the system produce more blood, open the lower digestive tract, and clean the stomach. Plums are very useful in subduing excess Wind (Vata) and Bile (Pitta). They give strength to the liver and purify the blood by expelling toxins from the body.

If plums are pickled in vinegar, they make an excellent appetizer and help in digestion.

Plums are eaten dried or fresh. Dried plums are a medicine for fever. Raw sour plums are not good to eat. (Plums are sour only when they are unripe. If an unripe plum is kept for a few days, it becomes ripe and then may be eaten).

Cooked in vegetable dishes, sour plums are healthy to eat, their sour taste providing a good substitute for dried pomegranate seeds.

Pomegranates
Sweet, sour, astringent; Cooling; Increase Wind

Pomegranates subdue Bile (Pitta) and Mucus (Kapha). They are palatable and unctuous. Pomegranates are found in two varieties:

❖ Sweet with small seeds
❖ Sweet/sour with large seeds.

Both varieties are good for one's health. It is recommended, though, that only the sweet variety be used for eating fresh. The sweet/sour variety can be sun-dried and then used as a spice to lend sour taste to foods and vegetables. The sweet variety is cooling and has a cold and wet effect. The sweet/sour variety is cold and dry.

Sweet pomegranates cure dysentery, diarrhea, vomiting, dyspepsia, and heartburn. They cleanse the mouth, throat, stomach, and heart; they increase semen, purify the blood, remove restlessness, and quench thirst.

One pomegranate a day is more than adequate. Seeds should be swallowed whole and never chewed. In cases where heat has increased in the body, both varieties of pomegranate will provide a cure. If taken in excess, pomegranates create constipation.

Raisins
Sweet, sour; Cooling;
Increase Wind

Raisins made from the best type of sweet, sun-dried grapes are recommended. Not all grapes make good raisins. The high nutritive value of raisins has made them popular. Their sugar content is about eight times that of fresh grapes, and the quality of the sugar is as good. Raisins are the richest source of glucose, which is readily assimilated into the blood, producing the heat and energy that sustains physical existence.

Glucose is used by the brain to activate the electromagnetic energy in the body. It is, therefore, a life-substance that is regularly consumed by the body. While grapes are not available everywhere, in every season, raisins can always be found. Raisins subdue excess Bile (Pitta) and Mucus (Kapha).

Anyone who is weak, old, or suffering from a debility or disease in which the body slowly wastes away should eat raisins in some form. The iron content of raisins is easily assimilated and helps the system produce more blood. Because raisins are more alkaline than many other fruits, they maintain the acid-alkaline balance in the organism and provide it with more stamina and vitality.

Raisins are best taken raw with peeled almonds (roasted or unroasted), cashews, pine nuts, and pistachios. This makes a complete food, which provides plenty of nourishment for growing children. This mixture is especially good for students. It is not advisable to use peanuts with this mixture. Peanuts are tamasic in nature, whereas other nuts and raisins are sattvic (see chapter 6 for a discussion of foods and the *gunas*).

Raisins contain carbohydrates, protein, fat, and minerals, such as calcium, phosphorus, and iron. They also have vitamins, such as thiamine and niacin. Raisins are an excellent natural laxative. Those made from the large variety of sweet grapes (the seedy kind) are frequently used by Ayurvedic and Unani-Tib physicians for medicinal preparations. These raisins are boiled with milk and given to patients suffering from constipation, preferably just before they retire. Raisins made of large, ripe, sweet grapes (munnaqua) act as a tonic for the heart. People can fast on munnaqua alone for quite some time. Patients with certain chronic diseases can be cured by taking only munnaqua regularly for a specified period of time.

Raisins with milk or yogurt make a wonderful combination because they complement each other.

Raisins can be used in many ways: in curries, salads, breads, milk, yogurt, sweet dishes, baked foods, and confectionaries (jams and jellies, cakes, puddings, and pies). The best way to use raisins is to soak them for twenty-four hours, or at least overnight. They can then be mashed in a small amount of the soaking water and strained. The remaining water can be drunk as is, or added with the raisins to food.

The water in which raisins have been soaked overnight and boiled for 30 to 40 minutes is a powerful tonic. It may be given to people of all ages. Washed and soaked raisins may be boiled in milk as well as in water.

In the Ayurvedic and Greek systems of medicines, munnaqua raisins are used more often than the smaller variety.

Eating sun-dried raisins daily makes one healthy and energetic.

VEGETABLES

Arwi Root (Taro)
Sweet, pungent; Neutral;
Increases Wind

Arwi is a root vegetable that is neither hot nor cold. It is unctuous and heavy to digest, but if digested well, it gives much strength. Arwi subdues Mucus (Kapha). People who are hot and dry in nature digest arwi without any problem, and for them it increases appetite. In cases of dry cough, arwi root liquefies the dry cough and expels the mucus.

Available at Indian and Latin American groceries, arwi is slightly constipating. However, if black cumin, red cardamom, ajwain seeds, or ginger are used in cooking the arwi, then it becomes a nourishing food. Ajwain seeds, in particular, make it less constipating. Also, the use of garlic or fenugreek seeds with arwi makes it easier to digest.

Red Beets
Sweet; Heating; Increase Bile

Red beets, although a root vegetable, are not tamasic in nature. Because of their sugar content, red beets are sattvic. Their alkaline nature and iron content make them a blood-producing food. Their heat-producing quality makes beets a good food for those who dwell in cold countries.

Beets are found in two varieties: sugar beets (white) or table beets (red). The sugar beet is not good as a food and is used only for making sugar. Table beets are used mostly in salads, stews, and soups. Sometimes they are added to sweet dishes for color. Beet tops are cooked as a green vegetable. Beets are excellent pickled in vinegar. Beet sugar, taken raw or cooked, is easily assimilated by the body.

Although sugar is their main constituent, beets also contain protein, carbohydrates, vitamins, and minerals, such as calcium, phosphorus, and iron. Beet tops are rich in vitamins; they are also a good source of calcium, iron, and potassium.

Those suffering from iron- or calcium-deficiency can eat beets and beet tops as often as possible. Boiled beets are not as nutritious as raw beets. Pickled or preserved beets are not as easily assimilated as fresh ones.

Bitter Melon
Bitter, astringent; Cooling;
Subdues all three doshas

Bitter melon, also known as *karela*, is bitter in taste. It cures mucus and gases, and kills worms in the stomach. Bitter melon is especially suitable for mucus-dominated individuals (Kaphas). It creates lightness in the stomach and is a diuretic. Bitter melon is also an appetizer and digestive. It cures diseases caused by disturbed bile. It helps cramps when cooked in ghee or oil. People suffering from excess mucus should eat it alone, without tamarind or mango powder. Others can eat it as a vegetable prepared in any manner. It is good for pregnant women and diabetics, because it controls the blood sugar level and reduces the amount of uric acid in the blood. Its juice is good for liver, kidney, and mucus problems. Bitter melon helps the liver purify the blood and is very good for pregnant women. It is available at Indian and Asian groceries.

Sweet Carrots
Sweet, astringent; Heating;
Increase Bile, in excess

Sweet carrots are hot and unctuous; their skins are bitter. Bitter and pungent carrots are dry and aggravate Bile (Pitta). Sweet carrots are a diuretic; they aid digestion and clean the stomach and intestines. Because of their sugar content, they are heat producing. They are high in calories. Sweet carrots are also rich in vitamins A and C; vitamin B is found in them in small quantities.

Sweet carrots cure constipation and subdue excess Wind (Vata) and Mucus (Kapha). They help people with heart palpitations. Sweet carrots increase the production of blood in the system, give power to the brain and stomach, and help in maintaining celibacy. They are, therefore, a sattvic food, suitable for brahmacharias, ascetics, and saints. They are rich in carotene, which is one source of vitamin A. Carotene assists the mucus secretion of certain tissues of the nose, mouth, respiratory, and digestive tracts. Carotene also has a beneficial effect on tooth enamel, protein synthesis, and vision—hence the saying, "Did you ever see a rabbit wearing glasses?"

Carrots are a rich source of calcium. A natural antiseptic, they keep the intestines free from bacteria. They are both a food and a medicine.

In cases of chronic diarrhea and colitis, carrots are a good dietary item. They also cure skin diseases. Fasting on milk and carrots alone for two or three weeks cures most chronic skin diseases. Women and children especially should consume plenty of carrots to keep their skin soft and shiny.

In India, carrots are used in many ways: as a sweet dish, as a fruit, as a vegetable. They are also juiced, and pickled in vinegar. Carrots are sometimes used in a raita (yogurt salad) and may be cooked with milk as in kheer (a milk dessert). When used as a fruit, carrots should be eaten raw.

While cooking carrots as a vegetable, fenugreek seeds can be added, or they can be cooked with turmeric and coriander powder. Carrots cooked in combination with cabbage, brussels sprouts, cauliflower, or potatoes are excellent. A *pulao* (rice pilaf) may be made with the above-mentioned vegetables. Carrots with green peas make a tasty dish and a highly nutritious food. Carrots remove uric acid from the blood and are good for ailments of gout and

SOOTHING VEGETABLES

Arwi root (taro), cooked	Subdues Bile (Pitta) and Mucus (Kapha)
Red beets, raw and cooked	Subdue Wind (Vata) and Mucus (Kapha)
Bitter melon (karela), cooked	Subdues all three doshas
Sweet carrots, raw and cooked	Subdue Wind (Vata) and Mucus (Kapha)
Cucumbers, raw	Subdue Wind (Vata) and Bile (Pitta)
Peas, raw (when tender and fresh) and cooked	Subdue Bile (Pitta) and Mucus (Kapha); Increase Wind (Vata)
Plantains, cooked	Subdue Bile (Pitta) and Mucus (Kapha)
Potatoes, cooked	Subdue Bile (Pitta) and Mucus (Kapha)
Spinach, cooked	Subdues Bile (Pitta) and Mucus (Kapha)
Sweet potatoes, cooked	Subdue Wind (Vata) and Bile (Pitta)
Tomatoes, cooked	Subdue Wind (Vata)
Turnips, cooked	Balance all three doshas

gallstones. As a fat-free food, carrots are beneficial in treating liver diseases. Carrots regulate menstrual discharge. Their use, however, should be avoided by diabetics and those patients who have excessive urination.

Cucumbers
Sweet, astringent; Cooling; Increase Mucus

The cucumber is regarded as a holy fruit in northern India. For the birthday celebration of Krishna (Krishna Janmashtami), every Vaishnava (believer in Vishnu, the Lord of Preservation) brings a cucumber for worship. It is a sattvic, light food. The cucumber belongs to the squash family and, in very small quantities, contains all the food substances necessary for the preservation of health. Thin-skinned, unwaxed cucumbers are best. Cucumbers contain protein, carbohydrates, fat, and vitamins, such as thiamine, riboflavin, ascorbic acid, nicotinic acid, and vitamin A; they also contain minerals, such as calcium, phosphorus, and iron.

The cucumber is cooling, calming, and refreshing. It works magically on restlessness caused by heat; its juice gives instantaneous relief to any burning sensation in the stomach. Cucumbers counteract hyperacidity, and gastric or duodenal ulcers. Whether in the form of juice or cooked as soup, cucumbers can be given safely to patients who cannot digest even milk. While solid, raw cucumbers cannot be tolerated by patients with chronic stomach trouble or intestinal diseases like ulcers, they can easily digest cucumber juice or soup in small quantities.

Because it is an alkali-forming food, cucumber helps protect against acidity in the organism. Cucumbers cure constipation and are popularly used in salads, as well as in pickled foods. Cucumbers are also a diuretic and encourage the free flow of urine when eaten fresh and raw (with a touch of salt, if desired).

Cucumber and yogurt together make a wonderful dish (see page 188). The best way to eat cucumbers is raw, without any seasonings. Their seeds are nutritious and are dispensed in India by Vaidyas and Hakims. The seeds contain protein and fat and are used as a general tonic.

Both ends of a cucumber contain bitter-tasting chemical substances. For this reason, in India the top half-inch and the bottom quarter-inch are discarded.

Plantains
Astringent; Cooling; Increase Mucus

Plantains are large, green cooking bananas that have more starch than regular bananas. They are cold and unctuous and slightly mucus-producing. They provide strength, help in building tissues, and increase the body's production of blood and fat. Those with weak digestive power should not eat too many.

Available at Latin American and some Indian and Asian groceries, plantains cure excess heat and diseases of the blood; they are slightly constipating and an aphrodisiac. For women suffering from leukorrhea or vaginal bleeding, they are an ideal food.

White Potatoes
Sweet, salty, astringent; Cooling; Increase Wind

Potatoes are cold and dry; they tend to solidify stools. The main minerals in this starchy tuber are potassium, calcium, and phosphorus.

Before cooking, potatoes should be scrubbed thoroughly in cold water. If the skin is very thin, no peeling is necessary. When potatoes are stored for a long time the skin thickens. Since underneath this skin is a layer of potassium that will enter the potato while cooking, it is best to boil them first, then peel them. The potassium makes them easy to digest.

The starch in potatoes gives energy. Potatoes are an ideal food if cooked with fenugreek leaves or seeds.

If potatoes are eaten to excess by people who do not exercise or do hard labor, they can create diabetes, dryness of the trachea, and dry skin. There is also recent evidence that overconsumption of potatoes by pregnant women may cause spina bifida in the infant.

Potatoes are grown practically all over the world. Because of their starch, salt, and mineral and vitamin contents, potatoes have been a staple for centuries. Since potatoes can be stored for a long time, they are used in many different ways. Eating potatoes alone is not good—they should be complemented by grains, beans, yogurt, milk, ghee, or oil. Oven-baked potatoes are easy to digest and healthy. If fried in ghee, potatoes become heavy and constipating.

Spinach
Astringent; Cooling; Increases Wind and Bile

Spinach is good for everyone, except those suffering from colitis. Since it increases Wind (Vata), people of this constitution may eat cooked spinach prepared with garlic and fenugreek seeds. Delicious if cooked properly, spinach is rich in minerals and vitamins. It contains protein, carbohydrates, and vitamins A, C, and riboflavin. It also contains the minerals calcium, iron, copper, and phosphorus. Spinach has more vitamin A than any other green vegetable. Also, its carotene content is more easily absorbed than that of any other green vegetable.

Spinach is well-known for its iron and copper content. It contains a substance that stimulates the iron already present in the blood, which activates the formation of hemoglobin. This makes it a good food for people suffering from anemia.

Spinach stimulates digestion and absorption. Easily digestible, it produces very little flatulence. Its postdigestive action is alkaline. It is not advisable to eat spinach raw because it contains oxalic acid. Oxalate deposits help in the formation of stones in various parts of the body. Oxalic acid aggravates gout and liver ailments. Also oxalic acid combines with calcium in the intestines and passes out of the body, preventing the absorption of this important nutrient. For this reason raw spinach is not good for children. Steamed, however, the oxalate content of spinach is separated from its cellulose, and when blended with spices, such as garlic, fenugreek, tumeric, coriander, cumin, cardamom, cloves, black peppers, and especially nutmeg, its harmful aspect is eliminated from the body.

Spinach is a mild laxative. It is not suitable for people whose stools are already thin. However, for those who have problems with bowel movements, spinach juice, soup, or boiled spinach leaves will provide an immediate cure.

Fresh, green spinach should always be used when available. Frozen spinach is only for those who need its laxative effect or its iron.

Sweet Potatoes
Sweet; Heating; Increase Mucus

Sweet potatoes are far more nutritious than white potatoes; they contain less water and more solid food. Sweet potatoes contain carbohydrates and protein and are quite rich in vitamin A. They also contain vitamin C, which is not lost even when they are stored for long periods of time. Phosphorus, iron, and calcium are also found in sweet potatoes. Apparently, some traces of panthothenic acid (B_5) have also been found in sweet potatoes.

With all these attributes, sweet potatoes are a heavy food. Therefore, people with a weak digestive system, sickly people, and those whose lives involve a lot of mental activity should avoid them.

In some parts of India, sweet potatoes are taken during religious fasts. They are mostly baked or roasted in hot sand, but sometimes are boiled at a low temperature. Baked sweet potatoes yield the best food value and taste, as they become deliciously sweet when baked.

In India, people make many kinds of sweet dishes using sweet potatoes. One simple dish is made by mashing baked or boiled sweet potatoes in milk (after having removed the skins), then adding a paste of ground nuts and seeds, followed by a few raisins. In cold climates, a pinch of saffron dissolved in a tablespoon of milk may be added to make this dish even more palatable and vital. The addition of saffron makes the sweet potatoes beneficial for both sick people and those who do a lot of mental work. If an extraordinary flavor is desired, either a few drops of rose water or powdered green cardamom seeds can be added. If a sweeter dish is desired, honey or raw sugar can be added. This is a delicious and easily digestible sweet food.

Sweet potatoes can be stored safely in a root cellar without suffering nutritional loss. Their sweetness increases in storage.

Tomatoes
Sweet, sour; Heating;
Increase Mucus

Tomatoes have become very popular in recent times. For the past 100 years, tomatoes have occupied an important place on the table because of their high vitamin content and the variety of acids they contain, which have a beneficial effect on the human organism. Tomatoes are a source of vitamins A, B, and C. The vitamin-A content is not destroyed through drying, and tomatoes actually contain more vitamin A than butter made from cow's milk. The high acid content preserves the vitamin C in tomatoes when they cook.

Because of the citric and malic acids they contain, tomatoes have a sour taste. The acids in tomatoes increase the alkaline content of the blood, which is nourishing for the blood.

Tomatoes contain carbohydrates in the form of invert sugar, which is easily assimilated. Due to their high vitamin content, tomatoes are a tonic. Tomatoes are a vegetable that increase longevity. Because of the starch content of tomatoes, those who wish to reduce should include them in large quantities in their diet. They are good for patients

suffering from diabetes. If taken raw, tomatoes are a mild laxative and are beneficial for sufferers of chronic constipation.

It is advisable to eat tomatoes when they are ripe. Green tomatoes are not harmful, but some people suspect the presence of oxalic acid, a substance never present in ripe tomatoes. Another consideration is that riboflavin is completely absent in green tomatoes. So, one should not pick green tomatoes from the plant but should wait until they start to ripen and change color. Tomatoes grown in open fields contain more vitamin A than those grown in a greenhouse or in a shaded area.

Good-looking, smooth, thin-skinned tomatoes can be eaten raw. People like to use tomatoes in curries, salads, fruit salads, soups, and with legumes and pulses. In northern India tomatoes are used in basic masalas (spice mixtures) because they add flavor and provide vitamins.

Turnips
Sweet, pungent; Cooling;
Balance all three doshas

Turnips are cooling and unctuous in nature. They purify the system and help it produce more blood. Turnips can be taken by people suffering from chronic dysentery and stomach trouble. However, in these cases they must be cooked with very little butter. A soup made of turnips can be given to patients suffering from fever.

Turnips are a delicious and healthful vegetable. They can be served often and are never harmful. Turnips are sattvic in nature because they have some sweetness. They may be used as a filling for *parathas* (griddle-fried breads). Young turnip leaves, a rich source of vitamins and minerals, are very popular in northern India. The roots stimulate the kidneys and are a diuretic. Turnips are prescribed for healing certain diseases, such as jaundice, edema, bronchitis, scabies, psoriasis, and eczema.

FLAVORINGS AND SPICES

Flavor involves the blend of taste and smell sensations evoked by a substance in the mouth. These sensations can be altered almost infinitely by altering the seasonings of the food. This is done mostly by the use of spices.

All spices are good for Vatas, if taken in the proper proportions and combinations, as in the recipes that follow. Vatas must take coriander seeds, which are cooling, only when they are combined with turmeric, a heating spice.

Generally, spices are not good for Pittas, with the exception of coriander, cinnamon, cardamom, cumin, fennel, saffron, turmeric, and black pepper (in moderate amounts). Kaphas can have any spice; especially beneficial are turmeric, ginger powder, garlic, fenugreek seeds, cumin, cloves, cinnamon, cardamom seeds, black pepper, anise, fennel, and saffron (in small amounts in soups).

Spices have a pungent aroma and are pleasant. Each has an appetizing and soothing taste uniquely its own. Internally, spices provide taste and change the chemical nature of the food; externally, each distinctive aroma creates an atmosphere that excites the appetite. Sometimes aromas are so strong they can be detected from quite a distance. Asafoetida, bay leaves, cinnamon, fenugreek leaves, garlic, and onion, for example, all have very appetizing aromas.

Some flavorings are so mild that their aroma can be experienced only when the food is served. Certain aromas make one think of salt-flavored food, and others remind one of sweet dishes. Flavorings also make foul-smelling foods smell good by removing the bad odors and changing the total chemical nature of the food.

The qualities of these flavorings should be very well understood. For instance, garlic and onions contain such strong chemicals that they taint the breath; this problem, however, can be easily remedied with the following recipe:

Combine 2 tablespoons roasted and 2 tablespoons unroasted anise seeds (if anise seeds are not available, fennel seeds may be used) with ³/₄ cup coconut powder. Add the powdered seeds of 16 green cardamom pods. Add 1 tablespoon finely powdered rock sugar candy, ground in a mortar with a pestle. Mix well and store at room temperature for up to a month in a covered jar. To cleanse the mouth and aid digestion, chew ¹/₄ to ¹/₂ teaspoon and swallow. This wonderful remedy destroys bad breath caused by garlic and onions or by disease.

Spices lend character to food and stimulate the taste buds. By producing more saliva, they increase the appetite and one's enjoyment of food.

Spices can be categorized as sattvic, rajasic, or tamasic:

Sattvic
Anise
Cardamom
Coriander
Cumin
Fennel
Fenugreek seeds
Rose water
Saffron

Tamasic
Garlic
Onions

Rajasic
Asafoetida
Bay leaves
Black peppercorns
Cinnamon
Cloves
Fenugreek leaves
Ginger
Mint
Ajwain seeds

Sattvic Spices. Fresh coriander leaves (cilantro, Chinese parsley) are delicately appetizing and are used in curries. Cumin powder is used to enhance the flavor of yogurt. It helps the digestion of yogurt and minimizes its mucus-producing elements. Cumin seeds have a piquant quality, ideal for flavoring dals, legumes, and beans.

Rose water subtly flavors water, making it more pleasant to drink; as well, it aids digestion and is beneficial to the eyes, heart, and nerves. Rose water can be used in all sweet dishes, particularly if they have a semisolid or liquid form. Rose water can be used alone or with cardamom seeds.

Saffron, the supreme spice, lends a sweetly succinct flavor to rice, yogurt, and most sweet dishes. It can be used alone or with cardamom seeds.

Rajasic Spices. Bay leaves, black peppercorns, cinnamon, and cloves are used in curries as flavorings. They also provide heat and energy to foods, which stimulates the taste buds and salivary glands. In turn, the glands secrete more digestive juices and the digestive fire is increased.

Cloves provide aromatic flavoring to rice and minimize its mucus-producing effects.

Fenugreek leaves give a good flavor to all vegetables and beans, especially to potatoes. Potatoes cooked with fenugreek leaves, and a touch of garlic or asafoetida, lend a soothing aroma to an entire house.

Ginger brings a pleasant bouquet to tea, and to all beans and vegetables. Mint adds a refreshing flavor to almost all foods. Although hot in nature, mint produces a cooling effect. Ajwain seeds lend flavor to wheat flour dough used for *parathas* and *puris* (Indian breads). They also aid in the digestion of wheat.

Tamasic Spices. Some people in India do not

use onions or garlic; many upper-caste Hindus—Brahmins and Vaishyas, for example—have not used these foods for generations. Even those who ordinarily eat onions and garlic avoid their use in religious feasts.

Anise
Sweet, pungent; Heating;
Increases Bile

Anise grows in abundance in all parts of India. It is commonly used as a spice in food. Often, after a meal, people take a mixture of anise, coriander, and cardamom with coconut powder to change the taste and refresh the mouth.

Anise seeds are light brown, green-brown, or yellowish-brown in color. Anise is sweet and pungent in taste and pungent in postdigestive action. An appetite stimulant and a digestive aid, anise also increases semen, cures diseases caused by gas, and soothes fevers and burning sensations. Anise is an anodyne; it quenches thirst, cures eye diseases and wounds, and removes mucus from the intestines. Anise is a wormicide. It also helps the spleen, cures diseases caused by bile, and relieves vomiting.

According to the Greek system of medicine, anise seeds improve vision. They are diuretic and a stimulant. Since anise seeds increase the body's production of milk, it is advisable for mothers to increase their normal intake during lactation. A paste of anise seeds applied to a child's stomach cures all intestinal ailments. Anise seeds are also beneficial in cases of chest and spleen disorders, kidney troubles, headache, asthma, and inflammations. Anise regulates menstruation and helps women whose periods have stopped for any reason other than pregnancy.

Anise seeds cure any burning sensations in the urinary tract. Being diuretic, anise clears urinary blockages; in cases where one has loose bowels because of mucus, indigestion, or vomiting, anise seeds are very helpful. Being an anodyne, anise cures pain in the intestines caused by mucus. For dry coughs and to cure mouth diseases, anise seeds should be sucked. Anise seeds can also cure venereal diseases.

Taking anise seeds in drinks during the summer is very popular in India. It is advisable to use them in food as well during this time, especially in foods that produce mucus or gas.

Asafoetida/Hing
Pungent, bitter; Heating;
Increases Bile

Asafoetida, also called Hing, is the milk of a plant that is found in abundance in Persia. Once solidified, the milk becomes a dried gum resin.

Asafoetida, which is blackish-brown in color, is available at Indian and Middle Eastern groceries. It has a very strong, sharp odor when it is ground. It creates a burning sensation when applied to the skin. Asafoetida subdues excess Wind (Vata) and Mucus (Kapha).

Ayurveda describes asafoetida as having a pungent and bitter taste. It has a heating effect on the system; it is lightly unctuous in nature and aids in digestion. Ayurvedic texts say it is a laxative and an appetizer; it increases the stomach fire and cures dry coughs, asthma, heart diseases, indigestion, worms in the intestines, lymphatic disorders, and tumors of the stomach. It regulates the menstrual cycle, cures ailments of the liver and spleen, gives strength to the body, and is beneficial in cases of paralysis, deafness, dizziness, shortness of breath, rheumatism, eye sores, and throat diseases.

According to the Greek system of healing, asafoetida gives power to the brain, liver, and nervous system. It helps the organism synchronize with seasonal changes, cures all kinds of inflammations, and increases the power of memory; it is also a wormicide.

Asafoetida contains an essential oil that evaporates quickly. When applied to the skin, it penetrates the pores, killing germs. This oil stimulates the areas to which it is applied and makes the body discharge all its toxins through sweat, phlegm, and urine. Applied to the throat and chest, it helps cure colds and cough. At the same time, it strengthens the system. In cases of severe bronchitis, asafoetida (a few drops of liquid extract in 1/4 cup of warm water) purifies the trachea and the lungs by first watering down the phlegm and removing the bad odor of the mucus. It then slows down the rate of breathing which takes away the cough.

In cases of nervous tension, when a patient becomes irritable, forgetful, pessimistic, moody, and depressed, asafoetida is reputed to be soothing to the nerves; it balances the rhythms of the body. Asafoetida is used by Ayurvedic and Unani-Tib physicians for all heart ailments, whether the disorder is palpitations, pain in the heart, angina pectoris, or "sinking" of the heart (as in depression or the literal slowing of the heartbeat associated with some heart troubles).

Asafoetida is often taken internally after it has been dissolved in a small amount of water for easy swallowing. Given at the time of childbirth, asafoetida helps the mother with delivery and, most importantly, helps to expel toxins with the afterbirth. Asafoetida cleans the womb and stops pain. Its use has also yielded miraculous results in cases of pneumonia and globus hystericus (the sensation of having a lump in the throat or difficulty in swallowing).

In Ceylon, asafoetida boiled in coconut water is used to cure snake and scorpion bites.

Bay Leaves
Sweet, bitter; Heating;
Increases Bile

The bay tree is found in the Himalayas at an altitude of 3,000 to 8,000, feet. Bay leaves contain the oils rutin and furocoumarin, which are stimulants for the skin.

Bay leaves cure heart troubles, stimulate appetite, and promote digestion. They also lend fantastic flavor and aroma to food. Bay leaves are bitter and sweet in taste. According to Ayurveda, bay leaves are hot and dry in nature and subdue conditions caused by excess Wind (Vata) and Mucus (Kapha). They work extremely well in cases of skin rashes and skin irritations, either taken internally, in the form of bay leaf tea, or externally, in the form of a paste made from crushed bay leaves. They also cure piles and diseases of the anus and large intestine.

Bay leaves are especially beneficial when used in food that is particularly mucus-producing. They cure indigestion, pain in the stomach, loose bowels, diseases of the alimentary canal, and coughs.

According to the Greek system of healing, bay leaves are hot and dry in the second stage of postdigestive action. They help produce wind (*prana*), increase longevity, and cure conditions of the tridoshas.

Bay leaves help expel gas from the intestines; they clean the milk in the breasts of mothers who have just given birth, and regulate menstruation. The smoke of bay leaves helps delivery in childbirth. Bay leaves cure stones in the kidneys or urinary bladder by breaking them down so that they can be expelled. Bay leaves cure mouth odor caused by stomach disorders. If they are used in tooth powder, bay leaves will protect teeth from infection. They are beneficial for people suffering from jaundice and are good for liver disorders and intestinal troubles. Bay leaves cure madness caused by fear. Stammering will be cured and pronunciation will improve if a piece of bay leaf is kept under the tongue.

Bay leaves are also used for curing cataracts and partial blindness. A paste of finely powdered bay leaves is used in Ayurvedic medicine for cleansing the eyes and improving vision. Bay leaves are soothing and strengthening for the heart. They cure madness, tympanitis, venereal diseases, and winter depression. Finely powdered bay leaves may be used on salads or mixed into salad dressings.

Black Peppercorns
Pungent; Heating;
Increase Bile

Black pepper is a great appetizer. Easy to assimilate, it is a stimulant and diuretic. It contains the Five Elements in equal measure and stimulates the body to recycle chemicals and food already present in the system so that no new food is needed. The use of black pepper in vegetables and other foods helps digestion and creates a good taste. It is recommended that black pepper be taken with honey first thing each morning. Black pepper is light and dry in nature. It subdues conditions of excess Mucus (Kapha), destroys diseases created by gas, and increases digestive fire. Black pepper is a medicine for those suffering from coughs, asthma, indigestion, colds, excessive sleep, poor digestive fire, and constipation.

Black peppercorns are a wormicide and an anodyne. If taken in excess, they create aggravated bile. Black peppercorns aid in the digestion of fats; therefore, their use in foods cooked with a lot of ghee or oil is advisable. For bile-dominated people (Pittas), a modified tea recipe, made from five to seven whole black peppercorns, is good if taken with honey, milk, and other spices and used in small amounts. It is an aid as well for those suffering from abdominal trouble. The regular use of this tea with honey cures chronic dysentery. The tea opens the pores of the stomach and intestines; it increases fire and expels old deposits from the walls of the intestines. This tea also cleanses the trachea and expels mucus from the lungs and chest region. It is through the heat-generating effect of the tea (which increases circulation) that the lungs can discharge waste material and excess mucus. It also cures fever. To make regular black peppercorn tea, add fifteen peppercorns to 2 cups of water. Boil until the water is reduced to ½ cup and add raw sugar to taste.

Black peppercorn tea made without sugar is helpful in curing diseases of the throat and mouth. Rubbing it on the gums can relieve swelling. The tea also cures skin diseases.

A mixture of powdered black peppercorns with ghee, honey, or raw sugar helps cure all sorts of coughs, if used regularly. If powdered black peppercorns are administered with jaggery and yogurt at the onset of a cold, the cold will be prevented.

Excessive use of black pepper is harmful for students and for people who want to increase their power of memory.

Cardamom

Cardamom belongs to the family of ginger plants. Cardamom is one of the most popular spices used in Indian cooking. It is found in two varieties: Large black or red pods and small green pods. Both are available at Indian and Middle Eastern groceries, and at some specialty stores.

Large Black or Red Cardamom
Sweet and pungent; Heating;
Balances all three doshas

Trees of red cardamom are found in India and Nepal. Black cardamom seeds are an excellent spice and are used for flavoring curries and soups in every kitchen in India.

According to Ayurvedic texts, the large cardamom seed is aromatic, sweet, tasty, and appetizing; it aids digestion and is a stimulant. Black cardamom subdues Mucus (Kapha), Bile (Pitta), and Wind (Vata). It increases stomach fire and stops hemorrhaging and vomiting. Black cardamom also cures stones of the kidney and gallbladder. Warm and light in nature, it is a carminative and a diuretic. Large cardamom seeds cure diseases and pains of the anus and poisonous bites.

According to the Greek system of medicine, these seeds help strengthen the heart and liver. They induce sleep, improve the appetite, and cure swellings in the mouth. They also help to cure diseases of the teeth and gums. The black cardamom bark is used as a paste to cure headaches.

Oil extracted from cardamom seeds is aromatic

and a stimulant; it increases body fire and soothes the heart.

A drink made of cardamom and cantaloupe or honeydew melon seeds mixed together with water, honey, and lemon, provides a cure for kidney and gallbladder stones and for problems with urination.

Black cardamom seeds mixed with anise seeds cure all stomach troubles. To relieve a burning sensation in the stomach and alimentary canal, mix ½ teaspoon (2 grams) of rock sugar pieces with the seeds of 5 cardamom pods and 1 teaspoon anise seeds. Chew the mixture in small amounts. Large cardamom seeds taken with black salt will cure stomach pain and tympanitis.

To cure pain of the gums and teeth, boil seeds of 1 black cardamom pod in 1 cup of water until the water is reduced to ¼ cup. Use the mixture as a gargle.

Black cardamom seeds are good for the heart and are used as a tonic and aphrodisiac.

Green Cardamom
Sweet, pungent; Heating;
Increases Bile

The plant of green cardamom, which also belongs to the family of ginger plants, is an evergreen. It grows in shady places and a sea climate is the most suitable. Green cardamom is smaller than black cardamom and is used primarily in sweet dishes and drinks.

According to Ayurveda, the seeds of green cardamom are warm, light, and dry in nature. Green cardamom has a superb aroma—much stronger and more refined than black cardamom. Green cardamom stimulates Bile (Pitta) and soothes coughs (Kapha) and Wind (Vata). It cleans the mouth and the mind. Green cardamom cures piles, venereal diseases, kidney and bladder stones, skin rashes, and vomiting of any kind.

Green cardamom has been honored and praised in India since time immemorial. Green cardamom has always been used as a flavoring in sweet dishes and delicacies. In almost all Ayurvedic medicines that are orally ingested, cardamom is generally added to make the remedy more palatable.

According to the *Sushruta Samhita* and the *Vagbhatta Samhita* (also known as the *Ashtanga Hridaya*), two well-known Ayurvedic texts, green cardamom seeds cure problems of urination. *Bhav Prakash,* another Ayurvedic scripture, mentions that green cardamom seeds cure coughs, tuberculosis, and hemorrhoids. They also cure vomiting and serve as an expectorant, diuretic, and aphrodisiac.

According to the Greek system of medicine, green cardamom seeds are aromatic, diuretic, and carminative; they strengthen the heart, are a stimulant, and can cure headaches, earaches, and toothaches, as well as liver and throat troubles.

Green cardamom seeds also help weak digestion, are good for the stomach and appetizing, and cure nausea. The oil of green cardamom seeds is a miraculous remedy for night blindness and earaches. This oil can even cure scorpion bites.

Green cardamom taken after food with anise or fennel seeds and rock sugar candy refreshes the mouth, aids digestion, and pleases the heart.

Cinnamon
Sweet, bitter, pungent; Heating;
Balances all three doshas

Cinnamon is found in the Himalayas, Ceylon, and Malaysia. There are three main types of dried cinnamon bark used in Ayurvedic medicines and recipes:

1. The bark of the Chinese cinnamon tree, which is thick, very rich in oil, and khaki in color.
2. The bark of the Taj tree, which is grown in western and southern India and produces no oil.
3. The bark of the Ceylon cinnamon bush, obtained from its tender branches, is thin and reddish brown in color, aromatic, and rich in oil.

Bay leaf tree bark is also used as a substitute for cinnamon bark. Cinnamon bark is used in dry powders and pills; the oil is used in the preparation of liquid Ayurvedic medicines and creams.

According to Ayurveda, cinnamon bark is hot, light, and dry in nature. Cinnamon subdues conditions of excess Wind (Vata), Bile (Pitta), and Mucus (Kapha); it is a blood purifier, an aphrodisiac, and an anodyne. It cures skin rashes, burning sensations in the trachea, heart diseases, diseases of the anus, vomiting, loose bowels, mouth odor, and thirst.

Cinnamon oil is a painkiller. It stops bleeding and cures vomiting and loose bowels. It is also an antiseptic and wormicide.

Massage with cinnamon oil cures rheumatism and nerve pain. Cinnamon has an essential oil that enters the blood very quickly and helps the body keep an even temperature; it also increases memory. Cinnamon oil cures earaches and toothaches.

When taken as a spice in food, cinnamon excites the mucus membrane of the intestines, which increases the appetite. Being hot in its postdigestive action, it helps the intestines and stomach to properly discharge gases.

It can be added to milk, soups, and desserts.

For pregnant women, the use of cinnamon should be fairly minimal, because it may cause a miscarriage if taken in excess. It is recommended after childbirth to stop bleeding and to purify the inside of the uterus. Cinnamon also helps women with heavy menstrual flow.

Cloves
Pungent; Heating; Increase Bile

Cloves are the dried buds from an evergreen tree found in southern India. The plant is attractive and its leaves are aromatic. In India, cloves are used in worship and in Tantric practices. They are chewed with betel leaves and nuts, and they are used as a spice in foods. Cloves are included in thousands of Ayurvedic and Greek medicines. In other parts of the world, cloves are used for flavoring liquor, for aromatic baths, and in perfumes and tooth tinctures. Oil of cloves is used for relief from toothaches and sore gums.

Cloves subdue conditions of excess Wind (Vata) and Mucus (Kapha) and increase Bile (Pitta), if used in excess. According to the *Bhav Prakash*, cloves balance tridosha. They work directly on the consciousness, the nervous system, and the veins.

According to Ayurveda, cloves are sweet, pungent, and bitter in taste. They are heating in nature and are used in hot spice mixtures, like *garam masala*.

Cloves are an astringent, a stimulant, an appetizer, a rejuvenator, an anodyne, and an aid to digestion. They are good for the eyes, asthma, hiccups, colic, tuberculosis, and most diseases of the head. They quench thirst, help stop vomiting, and cure coughs. Cloves cure a bad taste in the mouth. They are a wormicide and cure fits of tympanitis caused by worms in the stomach or intestines.

Cloves increase white blood corpuscles, thus increasing the body's resistance to diseases, infections, and viruses. They stimulate the nervous system. Cloves alleviate congestion and make it easier to breathe.

Cloves are good for cleaning toxins from the body. When applied externally in the form of a paste or oil, they cure poisonous bites, cuts, pain, and swelling.

Coriander
Sweet, pungent, astringent; Cooling;
Balances all three doshas

Coriander plants, also known as cilantro or Chinese parsley, grow in abundance in India. They are quite small and grow to a maximum height of eighteen inches. Because it is used for chutneys, coriander is one of the most important of the masala spices.

According to Ayurveda, coriander is unctuous and light in nature and cooling. It subdues excess Wind (Vata), Bile (Pitta), and Mucus (Kapha). Coriander also increases stomach fire and cures thirst, vomiting, asthma, coughs, general weakness, and worms. It cures fever and is an appetizer.

Coriander leaves are sweet and astringent in taste and cold in nature. They subdue excess Bile (Pitta), cure fever, vomiting, and sore eyes.

The Greek system of medicine states that a paste made from coriander leaves cures inflammation caused by poison. Topical application of coriander paste (seeds or leaves) gives the impression of being hot, but in fact it cools burning sensations and only later becomes hot. For these kinds of inflammations, mix coriander with vinegar to make a thin paste the consistency of pancake batter and apply to the afflicted area.

The juice of coriander leaves will stop a nose bleed (which is sometimes caused by increased heat in the system) immediately. This juice, mixed with breast milk from a mother who has delivered a female child, relieves acute eye pain.

Coriander seeds are strengthening to the body and soothing to the heart. They subdue Bile (Pitta) and cure madness caused by excessive body heat, epilepsy, and fear. A paste made from coriander seeds and water helps rheumatism and relieves problems with joint articulation. Coriander seeds help in cases of excess Mucus (Kapha) in the chest, and help cure gases or excess Wind (Vata) and cramps. Coriander powder taken with rock sugar candy cures colic pain. Drinking a solution, made from coriander seeds soaked overnight, cures piles and neuralgia and stops blood in the stools. One-quarter teaspoon of powdered coriander seeds taken with a "peg" of any good liquor cures the stomach of worms. Coriander is specific for strengthening the urinary tract and in used in curing urinary tract infections.

Excessive use of coriander seeds and leaves reduces sexual power in males and stops menstruation in females. Too frequent use of coriander is injurious for asthmatic patients.

Cumin
Bitter, pungent; Cooling;
Increases Bile

Cumin seeds are popular as a spice throughout the world. A relative of caraway, this seed is yellowish-brown in color and is almost always heated to bring out its rich aroma. Cumin is especially recommended for growing children. Cumin is one of the few spices, along with black peppercorns and saffron, that creates an alkaline body chemistry.

In Ayurvedic scriptures, cumin seeds are called cold in action and light, dry, and slightly hot in nature. Being hot in nature, they are also a rejuvenator. They subdue excess Wind (Vata) and Mucus (Kapha). When cooked, cumin seeds have a sweet taste.

Cumin seeds are appetizing and aromatic and increase stomach fire. They aid digestion and kill poisons. They are beneficial to the eyes, soothing and pleasant, and good for the heart. They strengthen the uterus, cure fever, tuberculosis, tympanitis, and a bad taste in the mouth. They remove impurities in the blood and cure worms and piles, poisoning, and leprosy. Cumin increases milk in the breasts.

To cure a skin rash, add a small amount of water in which cumin seeds have been boiled to the bath water. Repeat this cumin seed bath several times.

Cumin seeds cure venereal disease, relieve urinary problems, and are a diuretic. Cumin also cures kidney and gallbladder stones and helps in all genital diseases. For piles, mix cumin seeds with water to form a paste the consistency of thick honey and apply to the anus for relief of acute pain. Eating cumin seeds with rock sugar candy also helps relieve piles.

The Greek system of medicine claims cumin cures gases of the stomach and gives strength to the liver, intestines, and kidneys. Cumin reduces mucus, cures constipation and swelling, and increases sexual virility. A paste of ground cumin seeds mixed with water cures eye sores, ruptures of the gallbladder, and kidney stones.

Cumin seeds stop hiccups when given with vinegar. They destroy worms in the stomach and cure nausea experienced by new mothers who are breast-feeding. The powder of roasted cumin seeds can be rubbed on the gums to cure a gum inflammation or toothache.

The oil of cumin cures scorpion bites. Cumin oil is quick in action, whether used externally or internally. Roasted cumin seeds with yogurt help constipation. The application of a paste of ground cumin seeds mixed with water reduces swelling of the testicles.

Black Cumin
Pungent; Heating; Increases Bile

Black cumin is found in Kashmir, the Himalayas, Afghanistan, and Iran. Ayurveda considers black cumin dry in nature, an appetizer, and an aid to digestion. It is beneficial to the eyes and a cure for fevers, coughs, swellings, head troubles, and leprosy.

Black cumin, available at Indian groceries, has all the qualities of cumin, except that it is a stronger diuretic. If the water in which seeds have been boiled is used for gargling, it relieves toothaches.

A drink made with black cumin seeds, honey, and water cures swelling in the uterus. The steam from water boiled with black cumin relieves piles; the smoke from black cumin seeds cures colds and relieves sinus congestion. Chewing black cumin seeds helps reduce inflammation of piles. These seeds are also used to cure hysteria and colic pain.

Fennel
Sweet/pungent; Cooling;
Balances all three doshas

Fennel has a taste similar to that of anise and is often used in cooking and pickling. While anise is an appetite stimulant, fennel is an appetite depressant. Fennel is an anticonvulsive, an aid to lactation, a nerve stabilizer, and an antidote to insect bites and food poisoning. It also helps expel worms and is used as an eyewash. Fennel seeds and anise seeds offer many of the same healing benefits (see Anise).

Fenugreek
Bitter, astringent; Heating;
Increases Bile

In ancient India, fenugreek was used as both a spice and a medicine. Fenugreek subdues excess Wind (Vata) and Mucus (Kapha). It prevents premature graying of hair and is slightly laxative in effect. Fenugreek is an appetizer, a carminative, and an anodyne; it also aids in digestion.

As a spice, fenugreek can be used with vegetables and in salads. It is beneficial to the lungs and intestines. Fenugreek leaves alone make a very good vegetable. They may be used fresh or dried. In northern India there is a tradition of drying the leaves and using them as flavoring for potatoes, cauliflower, cabbage, and turnips, as well as in various dals and with beans. They are flavorful cooked in butter or any organic oil.

Fenugreek is heating in its effect and, therefore, is an ideal food in cold climates. People who always feel cold and who have cold feet or a cold nose should use fenugreek, fresh or dried. The seeds of fenugreek may be sprouted and eaten for additional nourishment during the winter season.

Fenugreek aids those who are underweight and those suffering from weakness and tuberculosis.

Applied to normal skin in the form of a paste, with chick-pea flour, mustard oil, and turmeric, fenugreek makes the skin smooth and shiny. Fenugreek keeps hair dark for a long time if added to shampoo. It also cures constipation and helps those plagued with liver or spleen problems.

Garlic
Pungent, salty, astringent, sour, bitter;
Heating; Increases Bile

Garlic is more a medicine than a spice. It is called *rason*, meaning that it contains five out of the six *rasas* (tastes); only the sweet taste is missing. The sour and bitter tastes become more prominent in the garlic as it dries and ages. It is a Rasayan (a rejuvenator) and a complete medicine.

Garlic is hot and dry in nature. It is rich in sulfur and contains essential oils and vitamins A, B_1, and B_2. Garlic subdues excess Wind (Vata) and Mucus (Kapha).

Garlic increases and purifies the blood and is a diuretic and a stimulant. It relieves pain, increases appetite, helps digestion, and kills worms. Garlic is very helpful in relieving accumulated gas in the stomach and intestines. It is beneficial for the throat and has a good effect on the sexual organs.

Garlic also removes plaque in the arteries. It cures circulatory disorders, diarrhea, colitis, dysentery, typhoid fever, ulcers, dropsy, intermittent fevers, bronchitis, asthma, disturbances produced by climatic change, tuberculosis, and heartburn. Garlic stimulates menstruation. It is an antiseptic, a sedative, a disinfectant, and it helps toothaches. Garlic also prevents cancer.

In India, garlic is used for stings and bites—especially snake or dog bites. Garlic is a poison remover. It also prevents the skin from scaling. If a small clove is swallowed as medicine regularly first thing each morning, it gives vitality and virility, and rejuvenates the intestines.

Garlic aids the heart by helping the circulatory system. It cures irregular blood pressure and relieves constipation. It gives power to the eyes and improves eyesight and even cures leprosy.

Garlic increases stamina and strength and is good for flesh, fat, and semen. It prevents premature aging. Garlic should not be used in excess by bile-dominated people (Pittas).

Ginger
Pungent; Heating; Increases Bile

Ginger is grown in China and India and is a favorite spice of tropical and subtropical regions. It is available fresh, in root form, and dried, in powdered form. Both forms are good, but preference should always be given to fresh. It is hot and dry in nature. Ginger subdues excess Wind (Vata) and Mucus (Kapha).

If a little over 1 teaspoonful of fresh ginger is taken with a touch of salt before starting a meal, it will increase the appetite and help in the digestion of all sorts of foods. Ginger pickled in lemon is appetizing and also promotes digestion. It can be taken with or before food for about one week; after this time it will grow a white fungus and should be discarded. Ginger pickled in vinegar (see page 199) keeps four times as long. Ginger juice mixed with honey relieves congestion in the lungs and facilitates breathing.

Each food carries its own vibration and alters the psychic makeup of the one who ingests it. In ancient times, there was a tradition that if a Brahmin (a member of the priest caste) had reason to eat in the house of a *Shudra* (a person of low caste), he was supposed to chew and swallow two teaspoons of fresh ginger twenty minutes to a half hour before eating the Shudra's food. This would protect the Brahmin from any low vibrations contained in the food; otherwise, he would have to undergo purifications.

Flaxseeds
Sweet; Heating;
Increase Mucus and Bile

Flaxseeds are cultivated throughout India. They are heating and unctuous in nature. They subdue excess Vata (Wind) and reduce thirst, fever, and high blood pressure. When ingested, flaxseeds are very slimy and create viscosity in the intestines, thus helping stools to pass without difficulty. If taken in small quantities, the seeds create constipation. However, if 2 ample teaspoons (10 grams) are taken, they remove constipation. From 1½ to 2 teaspoons is an ideal dosage; this amount can be used to cure ulcers of the intestines and amoebic dysentery. Flaxseeds with husks are tastier and work more quickly in the system than the dehusked variety.

Ajwain Seeds
Pungent, bitter; Heating;
Increase Bile

Ajwain is a shrub that grows throughout India. Its seeds (available at Indian and Middle Eastern groceries) are widely used as a spice in cooking and in the preparation of Ayurvedic medicines.

According to Ayurveda, the seeds of ajwain are hot, dry, and light in nature. They are appetizing, an aid in digestion, and an anodyne. They contain the essential oil thymol, which acts very quickly on the system. Ajwain subdues excess Wind (Vata) and Mucus (Kapha).

In Sanskrit, there is a saying that ajwain seeds alone are able to digest hundreds of different varieties of grains. Ajwain seeds really have many good qualities; they have the same gas-killing quality as asafoetida; they have the power of black peppercorns to increase stomach fire; they have the sublimation power of cloves; and like cinnamon, they are a wormicide. Ajwain seeds relieve gas and spasms, coughs, piles, vomiting, and spleen troubles.

Ajwain seeds are not generally used for seasoning vegetables. They are used in the preparation of almost all pickles and in remedies for the stomach. Ajwain seeds are best used with dals—such as soybeans, garbanzo beans (chickpeas), *chana dal* (a split chick-pea)—and *dal masala* (a spice mixture). When cooking with any type of dal or bean flour, 1 teaspoon of ajwain seeds for every 2 cups of dal or flour helps to speed digestion and reduce gas. When making

Foods and their Healing Properties

bread, add 1 teaspoon of ajwain seeds for every 4 cups of wheat flour to enhance the digestive fire and aid weak digestion.

Ajwain seeds help cure fever, stomachaches, and problems created by overeating. They provide strength to the liver and spleen and cure dysentery. The seeds should be taken with foods that take a long time to digest. One teaspoon of ajwain seeds added to recipes using chick-pea and wheat flours will help these foods digest more quickly.

Ajwain seeds have an antiseptic effect on the intestinal canal. In cases of asthma, smoking ajwain seeds in a pipe relieves shortness of breath in the patient. The smoke of ajwain seeds is also good for relieving toothaches. Ajwain seeds are in Ayurvedic tooth powder.

Ajwain seeds are given to pregnant women in India because, in addition to their digestive benefits, they help cleanse the uterus. Ajwain seeds are also good for post-delivery fever.

The hakim Meer Mohammed, writer of the famous Unani scripture on medicine, also tells us ajwain seeds are a stimulant; they increase sexual feeling and virility and destroy gases.

A drink made of ajwain seeds helps paralysis and shaking. Water in which ajwain seeds have been boiled will cleanse the eyes and cure the ears of deafness. Ajwain seeds are useful in stomach, liver, and spleen disorders. They cure hiccups, vomiting, body odors, belching, difficulties in urination, and kidney and gallbladder stones.

If ajwain seeds are soaked in the juice of a lemon and dried seven times, and then ingested, they cure impotence.

In hot climates, the use of ajwain seeds in food should be limited to small amounts because of their dryness. In cold countries they can be used freely.

Pomegranate Seeds, dried
Sour, astringent; Cooling;
Increase Wind

Pomegranate seeds increase digestive fire. They are constipating and increase the appetite. These seeds should be used whenever a sour taste is required in food but not more than once a week. Pomegranate seeds have a smooth, oily nature. They subdue excess Bile (Pitta) and Mucus (Kapha).

Available at Indian groceries, dried pomegranate seeds are a good remedy for pregnant women who experience nausea, heartburn, indigestion, or restlessness in the heart region. Soak about 3½ ounces of pomegranate seeds in water for 2 hours and then rub them with your hands to release the pulp into the water. Strain and then drink the water slowly; within 5 minutes the discomfort will disappear. This remedy is best repeated three or four times.

Onions
Sweet, pungent; Heating;
Increase Bile and Wind

Onions are hot, dry, and unctuous in nature, in small quantities. Onions subdue excess Mucus (Kapha). They drive mucus out of the digestive tract and, especially, out of the stomach. Onions are an aphrodisiac. They sharpen the eyesight and generate milk and sperm.

Onions provide heat and, therefore, are good for the elderly and infirm and those who live in cold climates. They contain oils of sulfur compounds, flavonglycocide, vitamin C, and fructose.

It is believed that if one has white onions in the house a snake will not approach. This explains the presence and regular use of onions in many Indian homes.

Onions are tamasic in nature. In cold countries, they are essential. However, in hot countries they should be used less because of their heating quality. Their smell can be counteracted easily by chewing a few coriander seeds.

Onions regulate the stomach and intestines. They help in kidney troubles and inflammation of the trachea and cure anemia and dropsy; they also help relieve pain from insect stings, small burns, abscesses, and rheumatic troubles.

Onions lower the blood sugar level and are useful for diabetics. They subdue Mucus and provide the organism with virility and resistance. Onions are used as a poultice on boils that are not yet ripe. They are especially useful for diseases caused by cold. They are also useful for people who travel continually.

Saffron
Sweet, bitter, pungent; Neutral;
Subdues all three doshas

Available at Indian and Middle Eastern groceries, saffron is famous in India for its aromatic quality and healing power. It is widely used as a flavoring and for coloring sweets and delicacies as well as spicy curries. Saffron's special use is in worship: It

45

is added to sandalwood paste, which is applied to the forehead before meditation, for its calming effect on the nervous system.

Saffron threads are the hand-picked stigmas collected from the flowers of the saffron crocus. Saffron crocuses are almost three feet (one meter) high and grow in many areas of the Himalayas. Kashmir is famous for cultivation of good-quality saffron. Large amounts of saffron are also imported from Spain to India, mostly for making Ayurvedic medicines.

When real saffron is put in water and rubbed on a white cloth, it leaves a yellow spot. Artificial saffron leaves an orange or red spot, which only later turns yellow.

The regular use of saffron in sweet dishes and foods helps to keep the system healthy, especially in cold climates. Saffron especially subdues excess Mucus (Kapha). It is an antiseptic, a wormi-cide, slightly laxative, and a diuretic. Strengthening to the body, it relieves dry cough, pain in the head, problems of urination, and liver and spleen ailments. Saffron removes burning sensations; it is a stimulant and increases stomach fire.

In the Greek system of medicine, it is pointed out that the leaves of the saffron plant cure swellings and are helpful in cases of gout or joint pain. The pollen of the plant is called saffron. Bitter in taste, saffron increases virility in men and milk in the breasts of mothers. It is intoxicating.

In Tibet, saffron was very popular. It is good in cold climates because of its heat-producing quality. As a stimulant for sexual power, there is no spice equal to it.

Saffron's essential oil has an aphrodisiac quality. Whether used externally or internally, it provides instantaneous results. As with all essential oils, it works directly on the central nervous system. When saffron oil has been used in cases of madness and for diseases caused by a disturbed psyche or mental stress, it yields excellent results.

Saffron also regulates menstruation. If it is mixed with water to form a thick paste and then rolled into a lentil-size ball and kept in the genital area, it relieves menstrual pain.

The application of saffron paste on the breasts of a mother who has just given birth increases her milk. Application of saffron paste on the forehead relieves pain and tension; when applied to the chest, it gives relief from colds and pneumonia.

Tamarind
Sour; Cooling; Increases Mucus

Tamarind refers to the pulp from the hanging pods of the tamarind tree, native to India. Available at Indian groceries and specialty spice shops, tamarind is cold and dry in nature. It subdues excess Bile (Pitta). As a medicine it works very well. It relieves constipation. Unripe tamarind irritates the throat and creates defects in the blood. Mucus-dominated people (Kaphas) should not take tamarind. It is good for curing malfunctions of the liver, jaundice, or cholera. Ripe tamarind cures thirst and dryness of the throat in the summer. A cold drink made by soaking a little less than 2 ounces of tamarind in 2 quarts of water (with raw sugar to taste) is useful in protecting the system from heat. This drink also cures stomach ailments or an upset stomach.

In hot countries, tamarind is used in many ways. It has a high vitamin C content. It cures scurvy and is useful, therefore, for sailors and people traveling by ship, or for people living near the ocean or in damp climates.

Tamarind increases digestive fire and is a medicine for gastritis or colic pain. The seeds of tamarind are good for seminal diseases in men. For instance, if the semen is thin, or the power of retention is lost, or if a man suffers from wet dreams, these seeds are remedial. Tamarind concentrate is taken as a medicine for enlarged spleen. It also stops vomiting.

Excessive use of tamarind should be avoided, as it sometimes causes thin stools and spasms in the intestines.

Turmeric
Bitter, pungent, astringent; Heating; Increases Bile

Turmeric is hot and dry in nature. It subdues excess Wind (Vata) and Mucus (Kapha) and is one of the basic ingredients in *masalas* (spice mixtures) that are used for cooking vegetables and beans.

Turmeric purifies the blood and subdues accumulated gases. It relieves pain and kills worms; it cures jaundice, inflammation, skin diseases, itching, skin rashes, and diabetes. Turmeric removes toothaches and may be used as tooth powder with a pinch of salt and a few drops of mustard oil. It cures inflammation of the gums, and in India, it is applied to all sorts of inflammations.

Turmeric, like fenugreek, is used internally and externally. It purifies the skin and provides it with a natural glow and smoothness, if used externally as a paste made with chick-pea flour and mustard oil. For internal injuries, a small amount of turmeric powder should be swallowed, followed by a glass of milk. It can also be cooked in soups and other dishes.

SWEETENERS

Honey
Sweet, astringent; Heating; Increases Bile

Honey is smooth, dry, and heavy in nature. It subdues excess Wind (Vata) and Mucus (Kapha). Raw, unfiltered honey is the mixture of bee saliva, the pollen, and juice of flowers. Bee saliva contains an enzyme that converts cane sugar into fruit sugar and glucose. In addition, honey contains a small amount of soluble wax, which makes it superior in quality to other sweeteners.

Honey is considered a holy food. It is one of the five nectars in the holy drink, Panchamrit. Raw, unfiltered honey can be given to a newborn or to the elderly. In this form and in moderation, it is never harmful, always gives energy, and is assimilated by the body without taxing the digestive organs; it is a medicine.

Honey contains iron, phosphorus, calcium, sodium, potassium, sulfur, and manganese. Honey from small bees is nectar and in Ayurvedic medicine is recommended for use on the eyes. It cleans the eyes and is absorbed by them; it improves energy, cures diseases, and improves vision. In general, honey is good for the heart, throat, chest, lungs, liver, and, above all, for the blood, because of its alkaline nature.

If one fasts only on honey and lemon water for a period of three to six days, the body will become free from all bacteria. By adding honey to one's diet, one can enjoy a life free from bacteria and worms.

Honey keeps well for a long time. In the tomb of an Egyptian queen who was buried over 3,000 years ago, a jar of honey was found to be in good condition. It had not fermented or lost its natural flavor and taste. In medicine, however, Indian Vaidyas do not use honey that is more than ten years old. Fresh honey is preferred.

Honey is an incredible preserver; it was used by kings in India to preserve ripe fruits so that they could be consumed out of season. The stem of a ripe fruit was sealed with pure bees' wax, where it had connected to the tree branch; it was then put into a jar full of fresh honey. After six to nine months, the fruit would be as fresh as if it had just been plucked from the tree.

Honey is used as the base for many Ayurvedic medicines because it does not change the chemical balance of a remedy. Ayurvedic doctors usually mix medicines with honey before they administer them to a patient.

The process of assimilating honey begins in the mouth. Most of the honey is absorbed by the time it reaches the stomach; it does not need to reach the intestines to be digested. A medicine that is carefully mixed with the honey is immediately assimilated and enters the blood vascular system with ease. This helps the patient make a quick recovery. By carrying the medicine straight to the vascular system, without taxing the stomach, intestines, or liver, it helps to maintain the heart. This form of ingesting medicines is, in fact, miraculous for heart patients.

Honey taken with warm water or in large quantites works as a laxative. Patients with chronic constipation can benefit from an enema with hot water and honey. Honey with black pepper is a popular remedy for coughs and colds. Honey with powdered pearls and silver foil is given to heart patients. The silver foil is made of 100-percent pure silver. For improving appetite and digestion, honey is taken with ginger powder. If taken first thing in the morning with almond paste, it is a tonic for the heart and brain. Honey is recommended for growing children, weak and sickly persons, young adults, and pregnant women.

Honey should never be cooked or heated. By cooking honey, its natural, soluble wax is destroyed, its medicinal quality is lost, and it actually becomes toxic to the system. Nevertheless, honey is extensively used in cookery and in the manufacture of so-called health candies. Only raw, uncooked honey does not ferment in the stomach or produce gas.

Monkeys and bears are very fond of honey. Monkeys are afraid of being stung by bees and hence use tricks to get the honey. Bears quite happily suck the part of the comb containing the honey. The fur of bears is so thick that the bees cannot sting them anywhere except on the nose or in the mouth.

Raw Cane Sugar
Sweet; Heating; Increases Mucus

Jaggery, also called *gur* (in some parts of India, *gur* refers to date or palm sugar), is heavy, smooth, and oily in nature. It subdues excess Wind (Vata) and Bile (Pitta). Jaggery is obtained by boiling sugarcane until it partially granulates and becomes a thick paste. The paste is then allowed to cool and solidify into jaggery, which can be safely preserved. Neither the cane nor the juice of sugarcane can be stored for a long time; the juice will ferment within thirty-six hours, and the cane will dry out rapidly, so its sugar content will be lost. Necessity made people boil sugarcane juice, so they could have it available whenever needed.

Raw sugar made from any natural source is far superior in food value to refined white sugar. In villages in India, jaggery is valued much more highly than refined sugar. Jaggery is often used, for example, with roasted garbanzo beans (chick-peas) and peanuts, in milk and yogurt, and with bread and rice. Many candies, puddings, and other sweet products are made from jaggery. During hot summer days, jaggery drinks are taken to help maintain a balance in the blood sugar and to provide instant energy. Jaggery is good for the heart and liver and stimulates the body's metabolism.

Excessive use of sweeteners should always be avoided. A piece of jaggery after meals helps take away the feeling of being too full. For this purpose, wealthy people in India make special preparation of jaggery mixed with pure cow's ghee, nuts and seeds, plus a touch of cardamom seeds for flavor. First the jaggery is boiled to a paste, and then the other ingredients are added. The mixture must be allowed to cool and solidify.

In Vedic literature, one finds the word *sarkara*, which refers to a sweetener often used in the sacred fire ceremony, called *havan* or *agni hotra*. Sarkara is obtained by straining the molasses out of the boiled sugarcane paste. It is then refined with a seaweed-like substance found in local ponds.

Available at Indian and Middle Eastern groceries, jaggery contains all of the food substance of actual sugarcane. During the process of manufacture, jaggery is cleaned, but not refined. The quality of jaggery depends on its cleanliness, which affects its taste and color.

Jaggery contains protein and carbohydrates. A good source of vitamins A and B, it also contains minerals, such as calcium, potassium, sulfur, iron, and phosphorus. The molasses contained in jaggery is high in B vitamins, including biotin, and minerals, such as iron and calcium.

Sucanot is an organic form of granulated sugarcane juice that can be found in health food stores.

NUTS

Nuts are a storehouse of concentrated food material. They are a good source of protein, fat, and certain carbohydrates; they contain vitamins A, B, and C, and minerals, such as calcium, phosphorus, sodium, magnesium, and iron. Their use is essential for vegetarians.

The protein in nuts is of high quality—even higher than that in milk, meat, and eggs. This protein is as easily digestible by the system as milk. The oil content of nuts prevents them from undergoing putrefactive changes within the body. Nuts contain no uric acid, urea, or any other toxic matter. They are easily assimilated and hardly ever ferment in the stomach.

Nuts contain more fat than any other vegetable food. Because of this they provide more calories than any grain, legume, or fruit. Their taste is delicate and refined, and their food value is particularly healthy for young, growing people when combined with dates, raisins, figs, or apricots. They are slightly laxative in effect. The high nutritional value of nuts raises the nutritional level of foods they are combined with; hence, their use since the early stirrings of man in curries, rice, and sweet dishes. For good health, it is recommended that one eat a combination of nuts rather than selecting one or two favorites.

Nut Milk

After soaking nuts overnight and removing the skins, they can be ground into a fine paste. Nut paste is used in facial massages. By adding milk to this paste, a milk that is similar to cow's milk can be made. This nut milk is easily digestible and is good for very young babies and for the elderly. Cooked in cow's butter, it is especially good for women after childbirth. Nuts are also ingested this way by wrestlers and bodybuilders in India.

A curd of nut milk can be made in the same

way yogurt is made from cow's milk. When nut milk is brought to a boil and lime juice is added, the milk curdles and thus the "curd" is produced. This curd can be used in sweet dishes.

Nut Oil
Almond, cashew, peanut, and walnut oils are used for body massage.

Nut Butter
Nuts in the form of butter are ideal. Taken fresh, this butter is easily digested and does not produce much gas. Nut butter is best made from roasted nuts and should, like all roasted foods, be eaten as fresh as possible. Nut butter with honey is nourishing and at the same time cleansing for the system.

Nuts need to be taken in proper quantities, preferably after they have been soaked overnight, peeled, and ground. If not soaked, they should be thoroughly masticated. Digestive problems arise if nuts are not thoroughly chewed: the digestive juices cannot react directly with the nuts, which will be expelled from the system without having been utilized properly.

Nuts are very good to eat at breakfast time, or throughout the day, if taken as nut milk. They are to be included in curries or sweet dishes with dinner. They should always be taken at the start of the meal, never as a meal in themselves.

For those who do not do physical work, it is harmful to consume an excess of five ounces of nuts a day. Only wrestlers, bodybuilders, athletes, or those engaged in sports can digest more than this amount without trouble. For the average adult, five ounces usually proves sufficient. For older people and children, two to three ounces daily will suffice.

It is always good to take nuts in combination with other foods. Different kinds of nuts can be used with dates, apricots, and raisins in equal proportion; they can also be taken with milk, yogurt, cereals, halva, kheer, rice pudding, curries, and breads.

Almonds
Sweet; Heating;
Increase Bile and Mucus
Almonds are heavy and oily in nature and they subdue excess Wind (Vata). Almonds are a superior nut and a favorite of most people. They are delicious, nutritious, and vitalizing. Almond paste taken with honey is frequently served to children in northern India. For people who expend a lot of mental energy, almonds are particularly essential. Almonds are equally popular with athletes, bodybuilders, and wrestlers.

Almonds contain the best-quality protein and fat. They also contain carbohydrates, vitamins, and minerals, such as calcium, phosphorus, and iron. The presence of thiamine (B_1) in almonds makes them a nerve tonic as well as a brain food. Because almonds are free from bacteria, their oil prevents them from fermenting. This makes them one of the best foods. Almonds are free from toxins, uric acid, urea, and fiber. As the protein found in almonds is of the best quality, they are easily assimilated and digested. However, since their skins are difficult to digest, Ayurveda recommends blanching almonds before using.

Almonds are eaten salted, roasted, candied, or sugared. They are served in the form of a paste, butter, milk, or curd; they are used in baked goods, confectionary, sweet dishes, salads, and curries.

Almond Paste
The best way to use almonds is to first soak them overnight and, after peeling them, grind them in a mortar with a pestle or, if that is not possible, with an electric grinder. (Grinding edibles with an electric blender or grinder is less desirable than using a mortar and pestle because of the change in ionic composition that occurs. Machines generate positive ions, which deprive the food of its negative, life-giving ions. Also, almond powder made with a blender or grinder is not as fine as that made with a mortar and pestle. Rubbing the soaked almonds against a flat sandstone surface is ideal; marble is too smooth.) Slowly add drops of water or milk, in which a few threads of saffron have been soaked, to the ground almonds and stir to form a paste. This paste can be taken alone or mixed with honey. When the almond paste is taken with honey and a pinch of freshly ground black pepper, its nutrients are absorbed by the fine capillaries in the mouth and assimilated without going through the stomach and intestines. Almonds are the only alkaline nuts, and honey is the only alkaline sweetener. Thus, this paste creates alkaline body chemistry if taken first thing in the morning. Seven almonds taken this way provide more energy and nutrition than one pound of roasted, salted, or sweet almonds eaten after proper mastication.

Almond Milk/Almond Milk-Yogurt

To make delicious almond milk for one person, simply add the paste made from 8 to 10 almonds to 1 cup of boiling milk. Cool and add raw sugar and a pinch of saffron or ground cardamom seeds. This liquid can be taken alone or used in other drinks.

Yogurt can be made from almond milk as follows: Bring the milk just to the boiling point, and allow it to cool to body temperature. Stir in the yogurt culture, and set aside in a warm place overnight (say, above the pilot light on the stove). Almonds are easiest to digest in "yogurt" form. As an alternative, they can be ground and boiled; this form is also easily digestible.

Almond Butter

This butter is made by soaking almonds in water, peeling them, and grinding them to a very thin paste. Either roasted or regular almonds can be used for making butter.

Almond Oil

Bitter almonds are poisonous and should not be eaten. Their oil is very good for the skin, however; massaging the body with a paste (made from 1 tablespoon of ground bitter almonds, ½ cup chick-pea flour, and water) improves the texture of oily or dry skin and makes people of any age look younger. The oil of bitter almonds is generally used in cosmetics for its scent and rejuvenating quality.

Consumption of more than seven to ten almonds per day is not good for the average person. If almonds are eaten raw, they should be taken with other nuts and with dried fruits such as figs, raisins, and apricots.

Cashews
Sweet; Heating;
Increase Bile and Mucus

Cashews are heavy and oily in nature; they subdue excess Wind (Vata). Several hundred years ago the cashew nut was brought to India from South America. Crops now grow in abundance in India's coastal areas. Cashews are the second most nutritious and popular nut, after almonds.

Cashews are sattvic in nature and rich in nutritional value. Up to 3½ ounces of cashew nuts in one day can be taken safely by persons enjoying good health. In addition to containing protein and

carbohydrates, they contain B vitamins—such as thiamine, niacin, carotene, and riboflavin—and minerals, such as calcium, phosphorus, magnesium, and iron. This rich combination of nutrients makes them an ideal food for everyone, especially those suffering from weight-loss, anemia, and general weakness. For anemia, soak washed raisins and cashews, in equal proportion by weight, overnight in water. Grind them and add some of the soaking water to make a paste to be spread on toasted breads or to be eaten alone. The remainder of the soaking water can be used to extend the paste into a cashew-raisin milk, if desired.

Cashew oil is superior to olive oil. It can be used in salads, for cooking, and for body massage.

Cashew Nut Milk

Cashews are best when rendered into nut milk (see description under Almonds). Made to the consistency of cow's milk, cashew milk may be taken as is or with honey. Cashew milk also can be converted into yogurt, which is good for the intestines, or used in sweet dishes or curries.

One can drink cashew milk or eat the nuts in a mixture of almonds, walnuts, or pine nuts combined with raisins, dates, figs, or dried apricots. These combinations increase the nutritional value of cashew nuts.

Pistachios
Sweet; Heating; Increase Wind and Bile

Pistachios are cold in nature and subdue excess Mucus (Kapha). Pistachio nuts are prized and sought after for their color, taste, and flavor. They are regarded as having high food value. A storehouse of valuable substances, they contain protein, fat, and carbohydrates; they also contain vitamins A and B, and minerals, such as calcium, phosphorus, and iron.

Pistachios aid in the production of blood. Their iron and thiamine (B_1) contents serve as a nerve tonic. Vaidyas and Hakims prescribe pistachios for patients suffering from anemia, debility, nervousness, heart trouble, low blood pressure, and many other afflictions related to the blood and nervous systems.

Pistachios are commonly used to revitalize and rejuvenate the system. They are eaten raw with other nuts and raisins by bodybuilders and wrestlers. They are used to enhance certain dishes—ice cream, puddings, confectionaries, pulaos, and curries—making them somewhat expensive. They are also eaten roasted and salted. Pistachios are best taken in milk form (see description under Almonds and Cashews). Pistachio butter is very good. In all sweet forms, pistachios are sattvic.

Pistachios should be used in moderation. Consumption of more than a handful a day may cause digestive problems. Pistachio protein is better than that of meat or milk; if finely ground or thoroughly masticated, pistachios are more easily digestible.

Pistachio oil is superior to olive oil. Although not commonly extracted, it is sometimes used in medicines.

Walnuts
Sweet and astringent; Heating;
Increase Mucus and Bile

Walnuts are heavy and dry in nature; they subdue excess Wind (Vata) in the system. Walnuts are best consumed in small quantities. Five to seven walnuts at a time are more than enough for one individual. If taken in excess, walnuts will stimulate bile and create indigestion, small pimples in the mouth, and irritation in the throat. If taken in small quantities, walnuts are good for the nervous system, the brain, and the body in general. They provide energy and alertness.

FOODS AND THE THREE DOSHAS

Wind-producing	Broccoli, Corn (flakes and meal), Lemons, Parsley, Salt, Squash, Tea
Bile-producing	Celery, Chocolate, Coffee, Curds, Mint, Onions, Parsnips, Peanuts, Peas, Pickles (sour and hot), Potatoes, Pulses, Soybeans, Sugar (raw), Sunflower seeds, Vinegar, Walnuts, Wheat
Mucus-producing	Avocado, Cabbage, Cauliflower, Escarole, Grapefruit, Greens, Honey, Kelp, Kohlrabi, Lettuce, Milk (bottled), Mushrooms, Pears, Persimmons, Rice, Spinach, Swiss chard, Tomatoes, Turnips
Wind- and Bile-producing	Banana
Wind- and Mucus-producing	Beets, Carrots, Chestnuts, Corn, Cream cheese, Dates, Grapes, Oatmeal, Olives (ripe)
Bile- and Mucus-producing	Endive, Sugar (refined)
Tridosha-producing	Cream, Milk (fresh, whole)

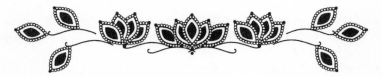

Chapter Four

GUIDELINES FOR PREPARING AND EATING FOODS

VIBRATIONS

Vibrations can be described as the subtle frequencies generated by the behavioral patterns and psychic makeup of an individual. Sometimes vibrations are so powerful that one can feel them from a distance; sometimes they are so weak that one must use touch to feel another person's frequencies.

By staying in a particular state of consciousness for a long time, one generates vibrations that can be felt from a distance. Sometimes people who are physically beautiful and who possess intellect and knowledge have vibrations that, for some reason, are disturbing. Conversely, some unattractive and uninformed people provide enjoyable company.

It is not beauty or knowledge that affects and influences others, but rather it is one's vibrations. Some seemingly angry and quick-tempered people draw others to them, while some silent and sweet-spoken persons can have very disturbing vibrations. Often we are attracted by exact opposites. But this type of companionship does not necessarily last, because only those whose vibrations suit us become our friends.

All things that exist, living or inanimate, have a certain vibration. Vibrations reflect the essence of one's being. Some vibrations suit our temperaments, some are neither soothing nor disturbing, and yet others are intolerable. Thus they fall into three categories:

Soothing (Positive)
Disturbing (Negative)
Neither Soothing nor Disturbing (Neutral)

Soothing Vibrations
All that we feel and express reflects relative truth; what is soothing to one person may not be so for the great majority of people. In the presence of soothing vibrations, one feels relaxed, inspired, and emotionally positive. These vibrations help one's growth and development, and give one encouragement.

Disturbing Vibrations
These kinds of vibrations either stop or prevent growth and development. They create restlessness and exhaustion. Such vibrations close one up completely and make one negative and discouraged.

Neutral Vibrations
These vibrations involve neither ignoring nor communicating. When communication does take place, it is on only a superficial level.

Although adequate scientific measures are not yet available to record all levels of vibrations, we do know that the human organism responds to vibrational frequencies very quickly. During this process the parasympathetic nervous system plays a most important role. Vibrations are registered by the sympathetic nervous system, but their interpretation is registered in the parasympathetic nervous system, which creates a pattern of vibration in the organism. This pattern vibrates the sympathetic nervous system and the hypothalamus gland receives a tone, a message from the brain. That message makes the endocrine glands active and thereby changes the entire chemical nature of the organism. This change in body chemistry creates mental fluctuations in mood and temperament.

Vibrations and Food

Thought vibrations are subtle and their effect on physiology, and thus on the human psyche, is profound and undeniable. Psychic makeup or temperament depends, as we have seen, on body chemistry. Body chemistry, in turn, is directly influenced by food input—"you are what you eat." For this reason, understanding the relationship between vibrations and food is of critical import.

Food is not just inert fuel for our bodies; it is as alive as we are. Ingesting food is a necessity, a compulsion. True, we are presented with great variety in foods—one can choose anything that is flavorful and easy to digest and assimilate. Yet the eating of food should not be treated as carelessly as it is today. It is common these days to see people eating hot dogs or some other fast food while walking down the street.

Large-scale food manufacturers do not concern themselves with the vibrations of their products. Every day people go to restaurants or bars where they sit and talk, and at the same time have a little snack and drink beer, coffee, or tea.

Many people have no time to think about food—they simply eat when they are hungry. They are not particularly interested in how, where, or what. Others are very particular about what they eat and like to explore new varieties of taste. Some people stick to a few easily available choices. Few realize the importance of understanding the qualities of food and the nature of their own living habits.

After many years, people eventually find out what suits their own body and what disturbs it. Very few, however, are aware of vibrations—from other people, from objects, from foods.

Whether we are conscious of vibrations or not, they do have their effect on us. Therefore, it is necessary to generate good vibrations wherever food is grown, sold, served, stored, or transported. Cooks should feel inspired and happy while cooking. Those who serve should feel happy while serving. Food cooked by someone who really likes to cook tastes quite different from food cooked by someone who is anxious. Both may be cooking the same dish, using the same recipe, yet the food will not taste the same. Just as human beings need care and attention, so does food. A cook who takes the greatest care will invariably produce a meal that not only tastes better but that is also better for the digestive system.

Food is made up of chemicals. Most of these chemicals are electrolytes. That is, they work as conductors and pick up the vibrations of the cook.

In India, it is traditional that the cook take a bath before entering the kitchen. This ritual serves two purposes: First, it makes the cook especially conscious of the job at hand, directing attention toward cooking rather than something else and helping put the cook in the right frame of mind to prepare food. Second, a bath cleans and purifies, calms and relaxes, and removes fatigue and depression.

Cooking is an art and, at the same time, a science. The art form involves an emotional relationship between the food and the cook. Cleaning, cutting, and chopping food are activities that can be performed with a sense of rhythm and relaxation. Cooking can be enjoyed as much as any other art—it becomes a creative act when it is done with complete non-attachment, with no emotional involvement. Like a clairvoyant, the cook receives intuitive messages—new tastes are born, new recipes created. The science of cooking requires a knowledge of cooking temperatures and food properties, food combinations, and medicinal applications.

In India, there is a tradition of not tasting food before it has been offered to God. Somehow, Indian people are able to prepare cooked food that contains everything in the right proportions. This is called "cooking by feeling." Food provides higher energy if it is cooked as an offering and eaten as blessed food.

When the sense of taste is deliberately not used, one's sense of smell, sight, and touch improve respectively. The energy that would have been concentrated in that sense will flow into the other sense organs, making them more receptive. I know a blind man who used to cook his bread simply by listening to the sounds it made during the process of cooking.

Making food for God to taste first, then accepting and eating it as *prasad* (food offered to and blessed by God); bathing and then cooking food while in the proper state of mind; meditating before eating—these practices force the cook to remain clean and pure in body and mind, and thus impart a high vibration to the food. Eating is worship; it should not take place in an unsuitable atmosphere. Food cooked or eaten in panic is poison.

The body is a temple. The individual consciousness that dwells in it is part of the cosmic consciousness. The body is a temple of individual consciousness. Each effort to make it pure and help its proper growth and development is a form of worship. Cooking, too, is a form of worship. The cook is a priestess or priest. Most chefs hired to cook in the homes of upper- and middle-class Indians belong to the Brahmin caste, the caste of priests. When food is cooked in a spirit of holiness, it is alchemy. Vibrations in the form of subtle charges blend into the food and make it taste divine.

The Sadhu and the Diamond Necklace

Once upon a time a very wealthy and religious landlord lived with his family and servants in a town situated on the river Ganga. They observed great austerities and lived according to the law of dharma. They were famous in the region for being humble and noble.*

One evening, in the midst of a great annual feast, a sadhu, or wandering monk, who was well-known to the landlord arrived. The landlord and his wife invited him to join the feast and stay overnight. Although the sadhu felt hesitant, he finally acquiesced. His room was in the very heart of the house, where daily worship was performed and where no outsiders could enter.

The next morning the sadhu awoke and left the house while everyone was still asleep. When the landlord's wife came in to tidy the room for morning worship, she found that the diamond necklace on the statue of the Goddess was missing. She informed her husband, Rai sahib, and their faithful servant, Chowdhry, of the loss. They looked in every place imaginable, but the necklace was nowhere to be seen. Finally, they gave up hope and sat down to discuss the matter. After much calculation, the astrologer concluded that the necklace had been stolen but that it would be found again. Hearing this, they all felt somewhat relieved.

Two days passed. Slowly everyone in the town came to know about the lost necklace. They were surprised that the

family had not reported the loss to the police or tried to find the necklace. But Rai sahib and Chowdhry had been furtively engaged in prayer, asking the Goddess to bring it back.

The morning of the third day, they heard a knock. The gatekeeper hurriedly reported to the landlord, "Sir, the sadhu has returned. He is weeping bitterly, Sir, and wants to see you."

"Let him come in," said the landlord.

When the sadhu entered the courtyard and fell to the ground crying, Rai sahib said in a very gentle voice, "What makes you cry, O holy one?"

"My karma," answered the sadhu. "Here is your necklace," cried the sadhu. "I took it."

"But why did you do it?" Rai sahib asked.

"Rai, I did not do it. How could I have done it?" inquired the sadhu.

"Then what happened?" Rai sahib did not understand.

"Before I came to your home the night of the festival, I stayed with a gang of thieves and ate with them," he replied.

"A dinner with thieves?" Rai sahib could not believe what he heard.

"For us there is no distinction and no discrimination," the sadhu said. "We dwell in a state of non-duality and believe all is one, all is God. With great devotion and kindness they asked me to stay with them and share their food, so I did. The next morning I bade them goodbye and went on my way. I walked all day and reached your place by evening. Then I ate your food, chanted, and went to bed. Around midnight, the food I had eaten the night before entered my blood and began to circulate in my body; that is what made me behave like a thief. I woke up in the middle of the night and removed the necklace from the Goddess, tied it in the scarf that I keep on my shoulder, and went back to bed. In the morning, remembering nothing, I left your home and started my day of walking. By evening, when I reached the ashram of my gurubrother he was pleased to see me but he said, 'Your face looks weary. You have done something wrong, Ramdass, I cannot look at you. You need purification.'"

"Suddenly I felt cramps in my stomach, as if I were suffering an attack of cholera. I vomited and shat all night. In the morning while bathing, I felt something in the cloth I keep tied on my shoulder. When I found the diamond necklace inside, I was amazed—how did this necklace come to be tied up in my cloth? Then, as in a dream, I remembered what had happened and called my guru-brother. When I told him the story, he said, 'I see, I see. It was the food!'

Jaisa khaow anna, vaisa bane manna
Jaisa anna, taisa manna.

As you eat, so is your mind;
As is the food, so is the mind.

---

* Ganges

54

"It was true. Hard work was required to purify that impure food. The effect of food stays in the stomach for about thirty-six hours. On the way here, I fell ill with a high fever, which purified my blood and my body. I have come to ask your forgiveness. Here is your diamond necklace. Do anything you want to punish me, because I am a thief."

Dumbfounded, Rai sahib, his wife, and Chowdhry forgave the sadhu for his actions.

INCOMPATIBLE FOODS

Certain foods are healthful when consumed alone but, when taken in combination with other foods, they generate harmful chemicals in the body.

Honey should never be taken with ghee or radishes. Yogurt should never be taken with foods that are hot in temperature. It should also not be mixed with milk, bananas (except when balancing spices are used), or tea.

It is not advisable to use milk with oil, salt, vinegar, green squash, radishes, bananas, lemons, oranges, plums, candy, sesame, and yogurt.

Milk mixed with water should not be used with ghee. Buttermilk should never be mixed with bananas. Also avoid the following:

Vinegar with sesame seeds
Honeydew melon with honey, yogurt,
    or water
Cucumber with water
Rice with vinegar
Meat with sesame, milk cheese, vinegar,
    or honey

Hot foods should not be taken after cold foods, or vice versa. Avoid cold drinks after taking tea, cucumber, honeydew melon, or cantaloupe.

THINGS TO DO
FOR HEALTHY EATING

- Sweet fragrances and the presence of gems and stones, flowers or garlands, or any natural decoration help to create a good atmosphere for dining.

- Food should first be offered symbolically to God, then offered to guests, old people, and children. Once the latter have been served and grace has been offered, the food can be enjoyed by the rest of the household.

- Wearing loose, fresh garments increases the appetite and improves health.

- Foods should be eaten while in a relaxed state. Washing the hands and face before eating creates a feeling of freshness and relaxation. Feet should also be washed, if possible.

- Eat only in a pleasing setting and with clean utensils.

- Eat only freshly cooked food, which is rich in pranic energy.

- Eat only when the right nostril dominates; drink only when the left nostril dominates. (The dominance of the right and left nostrils changes throughout the day. For instructions on how to change the dominant nostril, see *Breath, Mind, and Consciousness* by the author.)

- Eat only when hungry and after the previous meal has had time to be digested. Generally speaking, it is good to avoid eating until six hours after the previous meal. Avoid all between-meal snacks, including liquids (except lukewarm water). This does not hold true for children; they need food every three hours, especially when they take part in physical activities.

- Drinking water before eating helps one lose weight, but is not usually advised. Sipping a small amount of water during a meal helps assimilation and digestion. It also helps to keep one's weight under control and to maintain good health. Water dilutes digestive juices and acids, which help digestion. Basically, water should be avoided for an hour (or at least a half hour) before eating, and about an hour after eating.

- Eating should be neither too fast nor too slow: rushing will increase one's rate of respiration, while tarrying will make the food cold.

- Food should be thoroughly masticated so as to form a paste in the mouth. In this way the high-quality digestive juices in the saliva are transferred to the food. This enhances the process of digestion since assimilation begins in the mouth, not the stomach.

- Eat once or twice daily, as desired. Have a light morning meal and, if possible, a main meal before sunset.

- Taking food at a regular time each day is helpful in regulating the body's chemicals.

- Washing one's hands, face, mouth, and eyes after meals is good for the digestive system.

- Resting after lunch (not sleeping) and walking after dinner is helpful. If one cannot walk outside, one can take 108 steps indoors.

- Fruits, nuts and seeds, cream, yogurt, rice, and cereals or sprouted grains are ideal for breakfast or brunch. Freshly cooked breads, boiled or sautéed vegetables, curries, dal, and sweet dishes are good for the main meal before sunset.

- One-quarter of the stomach should be filled with grains and cereals, pulses, legumes, nuts and seeds; one-quarter with fruits and raw foods; one-quarter with water. The rest should be left empty to allow the free passage of body gases.

- Chewing anise or fennel seeds with coconut powder or cardamom seeds with the crystal of rock sugar candy after a meal encourages the secretion of saliva and thus the digestive processes in the stomach. The mouth becomes refreshed and one feels joyful.

- Regular use of milk, yogurt, cheese, or cream is good for one's health.

- More liquids should be taken during summer and more solid food during winter. Eating too little during winter is harmful to one's health.

- It is highly beneficial to cleanse the teeth and mouth after eating. Brushing, using dental floss, and massaging the gums help maintain a healthy mouth.

Things *Not* To Do
for Healthy Eating

- Avoid eating before sunrise and after sunset. If this is not possible, then yogurt, citrus fruits, and nuts should especially be avoided.

- No solid food should be taken before a normal bowel movement.

- Do not eat facing south, as this drains energy and creates anger; facing east is best. According to Hindu scriptures:

> To eat while facing East brings name and fame;
> To eat while facing West brings money and
>   prosperity;
> To eat while facing North gives deeper under-
>   standing and creates spirituality;
> To eat while facing South creates anger.

- Do not eat or drink while walking. There is an old proverb: I do not drink while walking, I do not eat while laughing—so how can I be a fool, old Man?

- Never eat unpalatable foods as this creates a resistance in the system.

- Cooked food should not be reheated; this renders it tamasic.

- Canned foods should be avoided or totally eliminated.

- Avoid eating extremely greasy or dry foods.

- Do not mix temperatures in the same meal: hot and cold foods should not be eaten at the same time. This is injurious to one's health and teeth.

- Avoid laughter while eating. Silence should be given preference over talking while eating. Hindu scriptures prohibit talking and stress the observation of silence during eating.

- Attention should be paid to experiencing the tastes in food and to enjoying the process of eating.

- Urinating after eating is good for one's health, while defecation after eating is detrimental to one's health. If possible, defecation should be avoided for at least two or three hours.

- Do not listen to meditative music after eating since this creates an upward energy flow. Laughter after a meal helps create a joyful mood and aids digestion.

- Do not sleep within two hours of eating; this disturbs the digestive system and the mind. Do not sleep without first urinating.

- Avoid tea or coffee for half an hour before or after meals.

- Avoid anything requiring physical or mental concentration for two or three hours after meals. Such activity disturbs the digestive system and the mind.

- Do not drink hot milk before going to sleep; lukewarm milk is good for those who have no problems with mucus.

- Indulgence in sexual intercourse after eating is hazardous to one's health.

CURES FOR INDIGESTION

Those who suffer from indigestion caused by a particular food may counteract their condition by taking another food.

FOOD	ANTIDOTE
Almonds	Raw sugar
Apple	Cinnamon
Bananas	Salt, Ginger powder, or Honey and cardamom
Bay leaves	Ghee, Garam masala
Berries	Salted water
Butter	Honey, Salt, or Raw sugar
Buttermilk	Lemon, Salt, or Black peppercorns
Carrots	Raw sugar (Palm, Date, Molasses, Sucanot, or Jaggery)
Cauliflower	Ginger or Garam masala
Chick-pea flour	Ajwain seeds or Pomegranate seeds
Coconut	Rice or Raw sugar
Cream	Mint or Honey
Cucumber	Ajwain seeds or Salt
Dates	Buttermilk
Dried milk	Salt, Lemon, Sodium bicarbonate
Figs	Almonds
Fish	Mango powder, Ajwain seeds, or Honey
Garbanzo beans (chick-peas)	Ajwain seeds
Ghee	Hot water or Lemon
Goat's milk	Honey or Anise seeds
Grapes	Rose petals or Anise seeds
Green beans	Garam masala, Ajwain seeds, or Salt
Guava	Ginger powder and Anise seeds (in equal measure)
Halva	Ajwain seeds and salt in lukewarm water
Honey	Pomegranate seeds
Honeydew melon	Lemon or Honey
Kidney beans	Rock salt or Cumin
Lemon	Salt or Sodium bicarbonate
Lentils	Ghee or Vinegar
Mango	Milk thinned with water
Marijuana	Milk or Ghee
Meat	Jaggery
Milk	Sodium bicarbonate
Moong (mung) beans	Sour foods (Pomegranate seeds, Lemon, etc.)
Nutmeg	Vinegar or Ghee
Oil	Lemon, Vinegar, or Pickle
Okra	Ginger powder, Ajwain seeds
Orange juice	Jaggery
Peas	Lukewarm water with salt
Pomegranate	Salt

FOOD	ANTIDOTE
Potatoes	Sodium bicarbonate, Salt, Warm water alone or with ajwain seeds, Garam masala
Pudding	Sodium bicarbonate
Pumpkin	Garam masala
Puris	Sodium bicarbonate, Salt, Warm water with ajwain seeds
Radishes	Radish leaves, Salt, or Jaggery
Red pepper	Honey or Ghee
Rice	Salt or Black peppercorns
Sugar	Lemon, Mango powder, or Pomegranate seeds
Tea	Anise seeds or Milk
Tobacco	Watermelon, Ajwain seeds, or Jaggery
Urad beans	Ginger powder, Asafoetida, Black peppercorns, Honey, Fresh ginger
Vinegar	Sweets
Walnuts	Pomegranate seeds
Wheat	Sodium bicarbonate or Anise seeds
Yellow split peas	Ghee, Mango powder, Lemon, Orange, Sour foods
Yogurt	Ginger powder, Salt, or Cumin

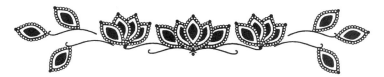

Chapter Five

FOOD AND THE CYCLES OF NATURE

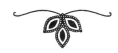

FOODS ACCORDING TO THE SEASONS

The energy patterns of the earth change according to its position in the solar system at different times of the year. These changes, which appear as seasonal changes, influence both the animate and inanimate matter on the planet.

In India, there are six seasons; in the West, four seasons are acknowledged. These four seasons repeat their cycle in an almost identical way each year.

Spring	March 21 to June 20	} Uttarayana
Summer	June 21 to September 21	
Autumn	September 22 to December 21	} Dakshinayana
Winter	December 22 to March 20	

These four main seasons are marked by two equinoxes—spring and autumn—and two solstices—summer and winter.

Each year on or about March 21 and September 22, day and night are of equal duration. On these two dates, the rays of the sun are directly above the earth's equator, as neither pole tilts toward the sun. These two days are known as the spring and autumn equinoxes.

On or about March 21, the North Pole starts tilting toward the sun, and it continues until approximately June 21, when it receives maximum heat, energy, and solar rays; this is marked by the summer solstice. The six-month cycle from March 21 to September 21 is called *Uttarayana* in Sanskrit, which means "toward the North" (the sun rises in the northeast corner of the horizon).

On or about September 22, the North Pole again is back in its right alignment and is not tilted toward the sun. But, after this date it starts drifting away from the sun. On or about December 22, the North Pole is at its furthest point from the sun; this is marked by the winter solstice. The six-month cycle, from September 22 to March 20, is called *Dakshinayana* in Sanskrit, meaning "toward the South" (the sun rises in the southeast corner of the horizon).

Ayurveda emphasizes the importance of eating foods that are appropriate to each season. Since the different seasonal changes aggravate particular doshas, it is considered beneficial during such times to eat foods that subdue those doshas. It should be remembered that, in India, the correspondences of the three doshas are distributed among the six seasons. In applying this system to the West, where there are four seasons, there inevitably will be some overlap. Thus the recommendations for early fall will overlap with those of late summer; those for late fall will overlap with those of early winter, and so on through the seasons.

Spring

Spring is a season of purification, a time to purify the system of the many toxins accumulated during the winter. With the coming of the new year and the accompanying change in the energy pattern, all living things start emerging from a long winter slumber. New leaves start budding on the branches. The landscape turns green again.

In India, this period is celebrated by a nine-day fast called the Vasant (spring) Nav-ratra. One may fast on two cloves a day, on lemon water or fruit, or on non-salty foods for nine days. The type of purification selected depends on the individual. This practice is still popular among Hindus today. People in other parts of the world also seek purification of the body during this time of year, either through traditional means or through methods they have devised on their own.

Mucus (Kapha) is aggravated in the spring, and the digestive fire becomes weak. During this season one should select foods from the following list:

Spring Foods

Apples, Bananas, Mangoes, Pears
Barley, Buckwheat, Wheat
Garbanzo beans (chick-peas), Lentils,
  Moong (mung) beans, Split peas
Asafoetida, Cardamom, Cumin seeds,
  Fenugreek, Honey, Mustard seeds,
  Oregano seeds, Saffron, Turmeric
Bitter melon, Cucumber, Eggplant,
  Ginger, Pumpkin, Radishes, Zucchini

The use of foods that are sweet, sour, oily, or heavy in nature, including yogurt, should be avoided. Salt should be used as little as possible. Urad beans are best avoided, as are potatoes (unless eaten with fenugreek leaves, cumin, ginger, or garlic). Foods that have a cooling effect, foods that produce mucus, and stale foods should be avoided.

Taking the scum of cooked milk (*malai*) with red cardamom and black pepper before going to bed helps one maintain good health during this season.

In Uttarayana (from March 21 to September 21, spring and summer), the sun is very powerful, and it makes the earth, and everything on earth, dry. The bitter, astringent, and pungent tastes become more dominant in nature. In cold climates, this is the most enjoyable time of the year. The blood becomes thick, from the heat and quick evaporation of water. The circulation of blood decreases. In hot countries, this season is exhausting and makes people weak and lethargic. In such climates people

need to drink plenty of water and sweet sherbets (a mixture of sugar and water) to maintain a balanced blood chemistry.

Spring, however, is the best time in Uttarayana; it is known as the season of Cupid (Kama, the Lord of sex).

Summer

Summer is a season of lethargy. The body naturally accumulates calories in the form of fat during the winter, as a protective shield against the cold. In summer this fat is automatically burned up; this process does not take place in the spring because Pitta is seasonally low. This burning produces a great deal of heat in the system, which creates dehydration. As this stored fat is broken down, the glucose content of the blood increases. Along with the amino acids, this glucose is eventually absorbed by the system to produce energy. While the fat is being burned up, the blood becomes thick and dehydrated. The vital fluids become denser and more sluggish, therefore taking in more liquids and sherbets becomes essential.

While in spring there are signs of new life everywhere, in summer everything is dry and most living beings suffer from exhaustion. In colder countries, people spend their time participating in summer sports. In hot countries, where people can barely walk outside at midday, sweat flows from the body as water flows from a spring. This depletion cannot be satisfied even by drinking large quantities of water. All natural salt leaves the body as sweat; the likelihood of getting sunstroke increases with the absence of body salt and glucose.

As the stomach fire lessens, the digestive power decreases. During hot summer days, Pitta (Bile) is aggravated; sweet, moist, and cool foods will subdue Pitta. The food choices that follow are excellent for a summer diet.

Summer Foods

Apricots, Bananas (in moderation), Berries
  (all), Bitter melon, Cantaloupe, Grapefruit,
  Grapes, Honeydew melon, Lychees,
  Mangoes, Peaches, Pineapple, Plums,
  Water chestnuts, Watermelon, All juicy
  fruits
Squash (all kinds)
Salads from: Celery, Kohlrabi, Lettuce,
  Radishes, Spinach

Turnips (root and greens), Watercress
Buttermilk, Yogurt

Shady places near mountains and trees are ideal spots to spend hot summer days. Seasoned (year-old) rice should be served, rather than new rice. Sweet dishes are also good. Lemon is excellent in this season, especially drinks made from lemon. Cow's milk or goat's milk, rose water, *gulkand* (a sweet, honey-like substance made with rose petals), and spring water (or water from a well) are ideal summer beverages.

Summer is the season to enjoy *raita*, a mixture of yogurt, fruits or vegetables, and spices. For instance, a raita made with cucumber and mint makes an excellent summer dish. Mint is ideal for cooling the system, and mint leaves can be used in so many ways. Powder from dried mint leaves is an excellent addition to drinks. Fresh or powdered mint leaves can also be used in salads. Cold mint tea is a good summer drink. When chutney made of mint (see recipe on page 196) is eaten with other foods, it helps stimulate digestive fire, which is normally weaker in the summer season.

Sour, pungent, salty tastes should be avoided during the summer. The following foods, which are dry and hot in nature, should be avoided: Garbanzo beans (chick-peas), Eggplant, and Urad beans; Bay leaves, Cinnamon, Ginger powder, Mustard, Nutmeg, and Turmeric. (The last spice can be used occasionally, but in small quantities.)

Anise, fennel, tamarind, cumin, and coriander are spices to be used in summer. A mixture of anise or fennel seeds, coconut powder, and rock sugar candy is also very refreshing (see page 37).

In India, people serve a delicious cold drink made from yogurt, brown or raw sugar, and cold water called a *lassi*. A special cold milk punch called *thandai* is popular among the wealthy and middle-class people of northern India. Fresh, green coconuts contain a lot of coconut water, which is very popular in coastal areas of India. Coconut milk, made from the meat of the coconut and water, as well as all nut milks, are excellent drinks. Foods that are dry in nature, whether hot or cold, should be avoided. Fasting on lemon and water is beneficial during the summer months.

Autumn

In colder countries, autumn is the season of changing colors; the weather is neither hot nor cold. Autumn is a time for activity—sports, exercise, and enjoyment. Less food is needed since sufficient energy is present in the atmosphere when the sun's rays are directly above the equator.

This again is a season of purification. In India, it is celebrated with a nine-day fast, much like the Spring Nav-ratra, called the Shardye (autumn) Nav-ratra.

As the North Pole slowly starts to drift away from the sun, the "night of Gods" starts. Preparations for winter begin. The body starts accumulating heat to fight the cold; this is one of the reasons Pitta becomes aggravated.

In Dakshinayana (September 22 to March 20; autumn and winter) the moon is powerful, and it makes the earth moist and wet. In cold countries, the beginning of this cycle is a good time. After December, when it starts to freeze, people need more calories to maintain their body heat. This season gives energy to people in cold climates; it is a healthy time for hot countries.

During autumn, foods that soothe the aggravated bile should be eaten. Sweet, bitter, and astringent tastes help soothe the Pitta dosha. The food choices that follow are ideal.

Autumn Foods

Barley, Maize, Rice, Wheat
Moong (mung) beans, Peas, Red lentils, Split peas, Urad beans
Cabbage, Cauliflower, Cucumber, Eggplant, Mustard greens, Squash (all), String beans, Tomatoes, Zucchini
Apricots, Bananas, Berries, Coconut, Dates, Figs, Mangoes, Melon

Red lentils, cucumbers, split peas, and zucchini can be used in combination with dal. Butter, milk, and other dairy products, used in moderation, help in maintaining health and vigor.

Winter

Winter is cold and dry in nature. In this season the sun is less hot and the wind is stronger. Wind brings cold and spreads cold; wind itself is cold and dry. Vata (Wind) aggravation is experienced inside as well as outside the system. Therefore, it is advisable to eat foods that are unctuous in nature during winter. Sweet, sour, and salt tastes help subdue the Wind dosha, Vata; ingesting food with these tastes will keep the organism healthy. Body massage with oil is a must in the winter. The oil pressed from black sesame seeds is ideal for winter massage. Mustard, olive, and almond oils are also very beneficial and heat-producing.

Winters in cold countries are very hard. To fight the cold outside and maintain body heat, a lot of calories must be consumed. This inner heat makes the blood thinner and increases its circulation. Since food is consumed quickly, more food is needed during this season than in any other. Heavy foods are more easily digested during winter than during other seasons. Winter is an ideal time to serve nuts and seeds with dried fruits.

Winter Foods

Buckwheat, Millet, Wheat

Garbanzo beans (chick-peas), Kidney beans, Moong (mung) beans, Red lentils, Split peas, Soybeans, Urad beans

Arwi root (taro), Bitter melon, Carrots, Green vegetables, Mushrooms, Onions, Peas, Plantain, Potatoes, Red beets, Spinach, String beans, Winter squash, Turnips

Butter, Buttermilk, Cheese, Ghee, Kheer, Cream, Milk, Rabri (clotted thick concentrate from cooked milk)

Papayas, mangoes, pomegranates, and apples are good for regulating the system in the winter. Honey taken with black pepper in the morning (see page 39) helps the system maintain a balance of the three doshas. Drinking lukewarm water helps digestion and elimination.

FOODS FOR EACH DAY OF THE WEEK

Eating a food of a specific color on the day that corresponds astrologically to that color or to qualities associated with it, brings the greatest harmony and benefit to the system (see chart on page 63). This system of food intake ensures a healthy rotation of proteins, vitamins, and minerals. The following selections will serve as a guide for the creative cook, who is sure to quickly add to this basic list.

Sunday
Do not use oil in food on Sundays. Yellow and red foods are best served on Sundays. Also, gram, beans, split peas, and buckwheat are recommended. (Dry and hot foods are best on those Sundays when one is fasting or ill.)

Monday
Rice and cold, watery (moon) foods, such as squash, cucumber, and cauliflower, are good to serve on this day. On Mondays one should look at oneself in a mirror (although this is a good practice each morning).

Tuesday
Jaggery (raw cane sugar), spices, carrots, red beets, red lentils, tomatoes, red cabbage, and sour foods are recommended on this day. Wheat is especially good on Tuesdays, but it may also be taken daily, especially in winter.

Wednesday
Coriander leaves, spinach, moong (mung) beans, mint, broccoli, brussels sprouts, peas, green beans, asparagus, and green cabbage are good foods to select from on Wednesdays.

Thursday
On this day, oil should neither be consumed nor applied to the torso or head. Appropriate foods for Thursdays are yellow foods such as saffron, garbanzo beans (chick-peas), cumin seeds, yellow fruits, and bread made from chick-pea flour or corn.

Friday
Neither citrus fruits nor sour foods should be consumed on Fridays. White foods, such as mushrooms, coconut, sweets (made with milk), fennel, fresh milk, and cream cheese, are preferred. On Fridays, foods of all colors can be incorporated into the diet.

Saturday
On this day oil can be used for cooking or in salads, or for giving a massage. The cook can also select from black beans, black-eyed peas, urad beans, eggplant, black poppy seeds, black cumin seeds, dark-colored plums, and black radishes.

Consuming a food that corresponds with the color of the planet on the appropriate day affords one a special and subtle strength.

DAYS OF THE WEEK AND THEIR ASTROLOGICAL ASSOCIATIONS

Day (English/French)	Planet	Planet Color
Sunday/Dimanche	Sun	Gold/Brown
Monday/Lundi Lunar	Moon	Moon Color/Pale Blue
Tuesday/Mardi	Mars	Red/Orange/Pink
Wednesday/Mercredi	Mercury	Pear Green
Thursday/Jeudi	Jupiter	Yellow
Friday/Vendredi	Venus	White
Saturday/Samedi	Saturn	Black/Dark Blue

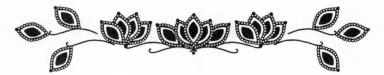

Chapter Six

FOOD AND CONSCIOUSNESS

SATTVA, RAJAS, AND TAMAS

Sattva, rajas, and tamas are not creations of the human mind but rather are three modes of primordial nature—pure, undifferentiated, universal Consciousness. Known as gunas, these three fundamental attributes present the natural evolutionary process through which the subtle becomes gross. In turn, gross objects, by action and interaction among themselves, may again become subtle.

Sattva, which means Essence, corresponds to Pitta.
Rajas, which means Activity, corresponds to Vata.
Tamas, which means Inertia, corresponds to Kapha.

By themselves, these three gunas are imperceptible. Being beyond perception, only the effects of their actions may be seen. By properly observing one's own physiology, one can note one or more of the three gunas actively directing energy into its respective channel(s).

The three gunas are explained clearly in the analogy given by Indian seers: Sattva, rajas, and tamas are three manifestations of the same essential substance called *Mul Prakriti*—or primordial nature—just as ice, water, and steam constitute three manifestations of the same substance, water.

In ice form, water, whose nature is to flow, loses its essence and mobility. It becomes static, confined to one form and one place. Ice is the tamasic form of the essence, water; the form in

which the movement of the individual particles have virtually ceased. Ice is water at rest.

In liquid form, the essence, water, is able to flow freely within the confines dictated by the shape of the container. Water is the rajasic form of the essence, water, and is the transitional state between ice and steam. To become steam, ice first has to become water and vice versa.

In steam form, the essence, water, is closest to its true nature, for it now fills whatever room it occupies and can go into every niche and corner. Steam is the sattvic form of the essence, water; it transcends the limits of gravity and form.

These stages can be called the three different phases through which all that exists passes. Sattva, rajas, and tamas can be seen as a tricolored braid: On the surface, one color appears dominant; yet, by observing the whole braid, one sees that the dominance is an illusion and that all three strands are ever-present.

Thus sattva, rajas, and tamas are not three separate entities, but rather three different modes or dimensions or frequencies of one single essence. One existence. One Reality.

The sattva-dominated person can look at any object and the past, present, or future of that thing becomes clear. The perspective is like that of someone standing on a high mountain peak, able to survey everything below.

The rajas-dominated person will try to fit any

object that he or she sees into a personal scheme of action, and he or she does so in terms of its present value alone.

The tamas-dominated person will be oblivious to the object, unless, perchance, he or she stumbles over it.

> Sattva is light, clarity, and understanding.
> Rajas is inspiration, activity, and pain.
> Tamas is doubt, darkness, and attachment.

One may choose to generate more sattva in one's life, or join the downward flow of energy into tamas, which finally ends in complete inertia—death.

Increasing sattva means generating more rajas and, therefore, experiencing more pain, more hard discipline, and deprivation of temporary sensual pleasures. Tamasic energy is consumed by the fire of self-discipline. Through the pain one experiences by generating rajas, the light of sattva dawns. This *tapas*, or "heat," leads to bliss, to the clarity of understanding one's own true nature, one's role in the universe, and one's role in the cosmic sport of the Divine.

One who understands the three gunas—their nature and their omnipresence—can recognize their operation within, during the course of daily actions and interactions. By keeping watch over one's actions and drives, one can, with the help of the knowledge of the gunas, assume responsibility for the development of one's own being. Keeping a watchful eye on one's habits—eating, sleeping, sexual—and on one's pattern of breathing, one discovers inner changes created by such things as food, clothing, colors, and sounds; by the cycles of the day and night and of the seasons.

By paying attention to these changes, one discovers that some foods are sattvic, some rajasic, and others tamasic. One understands what it is to feel light (sattvic), surged with energy (rajasic), or to feel dull and drowsy (tamasic). One will experience that events that produce attachment, doubt, ignorance, and sleep are tamasic in nature. One's own feelings are the clearest guide to the workings of the gunas within.

When sattva dominates, rajas and tamas are pushed into the background. During this time all inspiration to undertake action vanishes, as does the sense of attachment. There is nothing to do, nowhere to go, no job to tackle, no desire to eat

or sleep, no confusion. All that remains is knowledge, existence, and bliss. Sattva is light and capable of removing confusion by giving clear perspective. Sattva has the power of intuition, with comprehension beyond time and space. Sattva has the power of clairvoyance. Seers and saints come from sattva. The true nature of sattva is bliss. Sattva creates illumination, radiance, and tranquility.

When rajas dominates, sattva and tamas recede. At that time there is a great rush of energy, a surge of inspiration, and one has a distinct desire to undertake work and projects. Being a mediator between sattva and tamas, it is rajas that encounters both knowledge and ignorance. Rajas creates instability and one goes through cycles of positive and negative moods. Rajas is the power that activates. The nature of rajas is pain, which is an outcome of interaction and ambition. It is through rajas that the infinite becomes finite. The true nature of rajas is pain.

When tamas dominates, rajas and sattva become inactive. The tamas guna "stops"—it is the source of resistance and obstruction. Tamas is the energy form that creates doubt and confusion. Tamas is said to have a veiling power; it makes a snake out of a rope. Tamas makes one experience laziness, dullness, drowsiness, and attachment. In this state darkness and illusion prevail; delusion and ignorance become dominant. One does not want to go anywhere; one has no inspiration to work. Even hunger and sex do not provide incentive. The relational faculties become completely blocked and there is a wish for withdrawal, very similar to that of the sattva-dominated state of non-attachment, when tranquility appears. With tamas, however, attachment and ignorance are the dominating factors. The true nature of tamas is attachment.

The gunas are inseparable, yet interchangeable.

The Gunas and Self-Development

Self-development is the process of seeking and finding improvement over time in the state of one's inner being. Sattva, rajas, and tamas provide a very important key to this understanding. Without this key it would be impossible to find out whether or not we are really developing.

From sattva, to rajas, to tamas is the natural course of evolution in the visibly manifested world. Yet rajas can be used to convert tamas back into sattva. With our five senses, we have the choice of either flowing with attachment and desires ever downward into tamas, or of creating activity and moving upwards into the light of sattva.

The three gunas neither disturb nor contradict each other. Rather each one helps the other in solving problems, in evolving. Sattva, rajas, and tamas act together in unity and are present, in varying proportions, in everything.

Purpose of the Gunas

It should be clearly understood that there is no competition between the gunas: only one guna is dominant at a time. There are three gunas because energy has three modes. While energy is unfolding, it is going through a transition, which has three steps.

By using rajas to increase sattva, one can move against the natural gravitational pull and rejoin one's consciousness with the One, the Source, which gave us all birth. Thus the drop can merge back into the ocean. The prize for those who make the effort is *sat* (Truth), *chit* (Being), and *ananda* (Bliss everlasting).

SATTVIC, RAJASIC, AND TAMASIC FOODS

The main consideration when categorizing foods as sattvic, rajasic, or tamasic is their effect on the human organism. Do they create heat or dryness in the body? Do they create extreme cold? Do they stimulate the human organism—including the glandular secretions and the psychic centers (chakras)? Do they have an extended nourishing effect? What are the aftereffects? Are the foods readily digestible, or do they take some time and energy to digest? Do the foods disturb the doshas: Wind (Vata), Bile (Pitta), and/or Mucus (Kapha)?

Sattvic Foods

Sattvic foods are fresh, juicy, light, unctuous, nourishing, sweet, and tasty. Because these foods give necessary energy to the body without taxing it, they are helpful in achieving a balanced body chemistry—the foundation of higher states of consciousness, in which sattva predominates.

The psyche (*chitta*) is brought to a centered state by sattvic foods, because they bring readily digestible and nourishing food materials to the system. For aspirants of sattva and for spiritual growth and development, seasonal fruits, grains, and vegetables that are juicy, light, fresh, and sweet as well as easily digestible are the only diet. To eat only fruits, such as oranges, apples, bananas, grapes, and mangoes that are juicy (not pulpy), is ideal. If vegetables, grains, beans, and pulses are to be eaten, then wheat, cracked wheat cereal, bread made from freshly hand- or stone-ground flour (coarsely ground and with the wheat kernels), barley, moong (mung) beans, yellow split peas, rice, leafy vegetables, squash, milk, and butter are very good.

Wheat and barley are sattvic grains. As we have mentioned earlier, when cooked with excessive butter and spices, their sattvic nature is converted to rajas. Roasted garbanzo beans (chick-peas) are sattvic, but when eaten frequently, they produce gas and thus become tamasic. If garbanzo beans are sprouted and eaten raw they are sattvic. Fried moong beans also produce gas when eaten frequently and, therefore, give tamasic energy. Split peas are good if boiled with a little salt, turmeric, and coriander powder. They can be flavored with a small amount of cumin and asafoetida once cooked.

Fresh fruit juices from sweet, ripe fruits are the best sattvic foods.

Almonds, as well as sunflower, cucumber,

EXAMPLES OF SATTVIC FOODS

Butter, Buttermilk, Cheese (homemade), Milk, Yogurt

Barley, Rice, Wheat

Almonds, Black peppercorns, Fenugreek, Honey, Raisins, Raw sugar, Rock salt, Sesame seeds

Beets, Carrots, Cucumber, Green vegetables, Leafy vegetables, Moong bean sprouts, Spinach, Sweet potatoes, Squash, Turnips, Yellow split peas

Apples (sweet), Bananas, Coconut, Dates, Grapes (sweet), Honeydew melon, Mangoes, Oranges (sweet), Plums (sweet), Pomegranates, Watermelon

pumpkin, and honeydew melon seeds, are very nourishing. Almonds are rendered more sattvic when soaked overnight, peeled, and ground into a milky substance. In winter, a milky paste made from 7 almonds can be gently boiled with 1 cup of milk. Dates or raw sugar and ground anise seeds can be added, to taste. Ground seeds of the green cardamom pod or a pinch of saffron can be added to improve the digestion and give a pleasant aroma. In summer, water instead of milk can be added to the paste, which is then strained through a fine strainer. Anise or fennel seeds with cardamom and a little honey can be added. Although rose petals also can be added to these drinks, rose petals are best taken in cold drinks in the summer. After honey, raw cane sugar (jaggery) is the best sweetener and, like honey, it is sattvic.

The goat, sheep, water buffalo, camel, and cow all give nourishing milk. Of these, cow's milk is the most sattvic. However, four hours after milking, cow's milk becomes rajasic.

Kheer (rice cooked in milk) is sattvic. Fresh buttermilk and *lassis* (liquified yogurt with raw sugar) are also sattvic. The guna category for certain foods, such as lemons, black peppercorns, carrots, and sweet potatoes, is not so clear-cut. Because lemon is sour, it is not regarded as sattvic, but as a purifier, it is sattvic in nature. Black peppercorns are hot and dry but are considered sattvic. They provide energy to the stomach, increase the appetite, and clean and purify the chest region.

Carrots are roots and nearly all root vegetables are tamasic, yet carrots are sweet, cold, and unctuous, and they are easily digested. They cure excess heat in the body, help clean the lower digestive tract, cure diseases caused by gas and mucus, create more blood, make more urine, and thus clean toxins from the body. Carrots increase the digestive power of the stomach; they give energy to the brain and help in the maintenance of celibacy, and thus are classified as sattvic. Sweet potatoes, beets, and turnips are also roots, yet they, too, are sattvic and provide complete nourishment.

Mountain salt (rock salt) is sattvic and therefore recommended above sea salt which is rajasic.

Rajasic Foods

Rajasic foods are bitter, sour, salty, pungent, hot, and dry. These foods create sensuality, sexuality, greed, jealousy, avarice, anger, delusion, conceit, fantasies, egotism, and irreligious feelings.

Rajasic foods are tasty only if a taste for them is developed; otherwise, they are not palatable. They need to be fried and then treated with spices before they can be served. These are foods for people who wish to have material prosperity and who take part in the race of greed and competition.

We are living in a world that demands that we work to generate the mechanism of supply and demand. In all of our concerns, earning money is of considerable importance. We cannot spend all of our time in ecstasy, bliss, prayer, and meditation— we need to struggle for material existence. Nature is not kind everywhere. We need technical help to keep our homes warm and cozy. We have responsibilities and we owe something to society, which provides us with social security. Therefore we cannot afford to eat only sattvic foods, as did the saints and seers of ancient India. We need a certain amount of rajasic energy to survive. This is why we need spices and foods that sustain our energy level, enabling us to keep pace with the changing world. This does not mean, however, that rajasic foods are the only foods we must eat. We ought to keep a balance between the sattvic and rajasic foods, and try to avoid tamasic foods as much as possible. As rajasic foods produce excitement, we should take the necessary precautions to avoid overexcitement.

Foods fried in oil, sweets sold in shops, spicy foods, stimulating vegetables, salted bread, biscuits, sodas, homogenized milk, and all aphrodisiacs are rajasic in nature. Sattvic foods become rajasic if they are fried in oil, overcooked, or treated with pungent and sour tasting spices. Sattvic foods cooked in ghee are not rajasic, but sattvic.

Rajasic foods increase the speed of the human organism. *Rajas* is synonymous with motion and activity. Rajas gives sorrow, pain, and also involvement. Therefore rajasic foods create disease, sorrow, melancholy, helplessness, and exhaustion. In small amounts, liquor, wine, beer, coffee, and tea are rajasic. Taken in excess, liquor, wine, and beer (not tea and coffee) are tamasic. Drugs, such as marijuana, hashish, opium, cocaine, and heroin, are tamasic because they disturb body chemistry, dull consciousness, and obscure perception of reality.

Onions and garlic are blood purifiers. Ayurveda classifies onions as tamasic, but garlic, because of its medicinal qualities, is considered rajasic. Garlic is hot and unctuous. Excessive use can create dryness. Garlic increases longevity and produces muscular strength. It also increases semen and the glow of the skin and gives digestive power to the stomach. Garlic subdues excess Wind (Vata) and Mucus (Kapha). Bile-dominated individuals (Pittas) should avoid garlic. If it had a sour taste (thus giving it all six rasas) and did not have a bad smell, garlic would be categorized with sattvic foods.

Foods cooked in butter or ghee are sattvic, but when foods are cooked in oil they become rajasic. Raw milk that has been boiled for a long time acquires a thick consistency and becomes rajasic.

Red peppers, hot spices, pickles, oils, dry and fresh ginger, and salt are rajasic. Bread made with a pinch of salt is rajasic in nature. Foods that are hot in temperature while eaten, hot drinks, cold foods, and cold liquids are all rajasic. The temperature of food should not be greater than the temperature of the body and blood.

Rajasic foods create an unstable intellect.

Tamasic Foods

Tamasic foods consume a large amount of energy while being digested. They are dry, old, bad-smelling, decaying, distasteful, and/or unpalatable.

Tamasic food increases pessimism, ignorance, lack of common sense, greed, laziness, irreligion, criminal tendencies, and doubt. Tamasic foods create a severe inferiority complex and antagonistic feelings.

Foods that have been processed, canned, or frozen are tamasic. Foods that are cold and stale or that have been obtained by violence are tamasic, as are those that make one dull and drowsy. Incompatible food combinations—like milk and vinegar, or radishes and honey—produce tamas in the body chemistry. When hot and cold foods are taken together they become tamasic. Meat, fish, and eggs are tamasic foods. Candies, biscuits, and bread more than eight hours old are tamasic. Cod liver oil and shark liver oil, as well as hard liquor, are tamasic. Medicines that create dullness are tamasic.

By overcooking, foods become tamasic. Leftover food is also tamasic. Food contains prana, and this pranic energy is lost in food that is overcooked, overripe, or old. Dried milk, grains that create dryness, root vegetables (except carrots, beets, sweet potatoes, and turnips), and peanuts are tamasic. Indian breads—parathas, puris, and rotis—are rajasic but become tamasic about eight hours after they are cooked. All foods that create destructiveness are tamasic.

If one is interested in remaining alert and inspired, one should avoid tamasic foods.

II

The Recipes

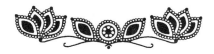

Chapter One

INTRODUCTION TO THE RECIPES

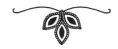

UTENSILS

In addition to the utensils usually found in a Western kitchen, the following are needed when preparing Indian food.

Wok (heavy)
Cast-iron skillet
Mortar and pestle
Rolling pin (thin, tapered)
Rolling board (round)
Tongs (wood or stainless steel)
Ladle or large cooking spoon
Perforated spatula or skimmer
4-Sided grater
Cheesecloth or soft cotton tea towels
Bread cloths (for keeping breads warm)

Wok

The shallow, round-bottomed Chinese wok is ideal because it requires very little oil for most cooking. It can be used for deep- or shallow-frying breads and breaded vegetables. Indian woks, usually made of cast iron, are also excellent because of the beneficial way in which foods interact with the iron during the cooking process.

Cast-iron Skillet

A flat-bottomed cast-iron skillet is ideal for making Indian breads on a gas or electric stove or open flame. It is also useful for roasting flours and spices and for all manner of general frying and sautéing.

Mortar and Pestle

By preparing spices with a mortar and pestle, we extract the best flavor and aroma from the essential oils, as well as the maximum medicinal benefit. Since a mortar and pestle are used in preparing almost every Indian meal, it is helpful to have various sizes on hand. The size of the mortar and pestle used depends on the quantities being ground. They are available in wood, stone, ceramic, brass, or glass. However, if this utensil is not available, an electric grinder may be used; a blender may be used for grinding dals.

Rolling Pin and Board
A thin, tapered rolling pin and round, wooden rolling board with feet are ideal for making Indian breads.

Tongs
These are used for removing large ingredients from a hot wok or for holding breads over a flame.

Ladle or Large Cooking Spoon
Tarkas—spice-infused oils made for dals, raitas, and other dishes—are best made with a soup ladle or large cooking spoon. A large ladle is also useful for serving soups and semisolid dishes.

Perforated Spatula or Skimmer
A round, perforated spatula or skimmer is invaluable when removing deep-fried foods from hot oil or ghee. The holes permit the oil to drain off.

4-Sided Grater
This tool is helpful when vegetables, such as carrots, beets, or turnips, need to be shredded for a dish. Each side of the grater offers a different degree of coarseness or fineness.

Cheesecloth
When sprouting beans or preparing paneer, a large piece of cheesecloth is a necessary tool. A large, clean handkerchief can be used instead.

Bread Cloths
Keeping breads in a fresh cloth helps keep them soft and warm. The best way to maintain the quality of freshly made bread is to place the breads on a clean cloth inside a pan, fold over the excess cloth, and cover with a lid. It is preferable to set aside certain cloths just for covering breads.

Measurements
Use level amounts for all units of measure: teaspoons, tablespoons, cups, and so on.

ABOUT THE INGREDIENTS USED IN THESE RECIPES

While a number of the ingredients called for in this book may be unfamiliar to the Western cook and difficult to procure from the average grocery store, many of them are obtainable from health food and other specialty stores, and nearly all can be purchased in Indian groceries. (For sources of supply, please see pages 256–257.)

For further information on unfamiliar foods and spices, please turn to the Glossary of Ingredients (page 253).

Ghee and Oils

Ghee made from cream or butter is ideal for cooking and frying. It is far superior in its properties and digestibility than any vegetable oil. It is a purifier that absorbs and expels toxins from the body. Even though it comes from an animal source, it is consumed by many vegetarians because of its beneficial effects. Ghee contains vitamin D, and since it does not have even a trace of milk solids, it can be stored for a long time without refrigeration.

Vegetable oils also are good for frying and cooking, although foods fried in oil are not as easily digested as those fried in ghee. Oil is rich in vitamins and minerals and, in combination with vinegar or lemon in salads, is beneficial for the body's metabolism.

When heating ghee or oil, it is advisable to heat the pan for a minute or two in advance. This heating process removes invisible dust particles and other residues that may be present.

In the recipes that follow, mustard oil is frequently called for because of its superior healing properties and distinctive flavor. It is available in Indian groceries and some specialty stores. Except where specifically indicated, sesame, sunflower, and peanut oils are all acceptable substitutes.

In this book, you will often see the phrase "until the ghee (or oil) surfaces." Once the vegetables and spices absorb the fat and become cooked, the ghee or oil is released; it reappears on the surface of the cooked vegetable or legume. This is an indication to the cook to cover the dish, turn off the heat, and allow the flavors to blend. The garam masala or other ground spices should be added just after the ghee or oil surfaces and the heat is turned off.

Ghee

8 ounces unsalted butter
4 whole cloves

Place butter in a heavy pan and melt over medium heat until foam rises to the surface. Take care not to burn the butter. Add the cloves, which will help in clarification and lend a delicate flavor, and gently stir. Reduce the heat to low and continue cooking, uncovered, until the milk solids collect on the bottom of the pan and turn a golden color. Remove any crust that rises to the surface with a large spoon and set it aside. Ladle off the ghee, taking care not to disturb the milk solids at the bottom of the pan. The solids can be combined with the reserved thin crust to use later for making parathas (griddle-fried whole wheat bread), or for serving with steamed vegetables or cereals.

Sugar

Sugar in any form is the most concentrated source of the caloric energy needed for the functioning of the body's electrochemical system. Sugar in the form of glucose fuels the brain, and along with oxygen, produces the combustion that generates life-force. It gives energy to whatever state of consciousness one is in at the moment the sugar is taken.

Sweeteners are mostly used to increase the palatability of foods. In recent years there has been increasing concern about their use because of adverse effects they may have on the bones and the liver. People are now becoming more selective in their choice of sweeteners and are using them in smaller quantities and with less frequency.

As a general rule, sweeteners (except for sweet fresh fruits and dried fruits, such as dates and raisins) should be avoided because the heat released by sugar can—when excessive—damage the liver. In small amounts, jaggery (*gur*) and Sucanat (*khand*)—both made from sugar cane—and other raw, unrefined sugars are not harmful. They also satisfy our natural craving for the sweet taste. These sugars contain iron, carotene, vitamin A, and thiamine. Traces of nicotinic acid (niacin) are also found in jaggery and Sucanat. Palm and date sugar (*tad-gur*) are also good sweeteners and can be used safely in moderate amounts.

The sweet taste after any meal helps fermentation and aids digestion. Ayurveda recommends having food with a sweet taste (*Madhur rasa*) at both the beginning and the end of each meal. But the ancient seers had no idea that man would invent white sugar (which is a slow poison that should be avoided completely) and use it freely to make sweet dishes and candies. There exists in nature a variety of sweet fruits, both fresh and dried, that can be used to great benefit before and after meals.

Flour

Wheat, barley, millet, corn, and rice flours are commonly used in breads, pancakes, cakes, and cookies. In addition to these whole-grain flours, buckwheat flour is also used in Indian kitchens, especially during the nine-day Nav-ratra fast in spring and autumn, when people avoid eating grains. Flour from pulses, such as urad beans, moong (mung) beans, garbanzo beans (chick-peas), and black gram, is also used quite frequently.

Flour from grains (cereals) is the cheapest source of calories, contributing as much as 70 to 80 percent of the calories in the Indian diet. Most of these cereals contain 6 to 12 percent protein. In view of their primary role in the diet, these cereals are also an important source of protein. Though they are poor in calcium, they supply the major portion of B vitamins, especially thiamine and niacin.

Garbanzo (chick-pea) flour and black gram flour (made from split black chick-peas, or *chana dal*, and commonly known as *besan* in Hindi) are good sources of protein and are used in combination with grains. This mixture increases the nutritional value of the proteins. These flours also make good binding material; they are sticky and enhance the flavor and overall food value of grains and vegetables.

Buckwheat, corn, and millet flours are less sticky. It is difficult to roll dough made from these flours, but this problem can be solved by adding a little besan or wheat flour. During the Nav-ratra fasts, buckwheat flour is used for making parathas and puris. To make the dough easy to roll, boiled and mashed potatoes, plantains, or arwi root (taro) are added.

Flour should not be stored for a long period of time. Whole grains contain pranic energy (life-force). They can be stored for at least one year, until the new crop comes to the market, without losing this vital life-force. Once milled, however, whole-grain flours hold this pranic energy for no more than two weeks and so should be consumed within this period. Enriched, refined flour should not be used at all. It sticks to the walls of the intestines and causes constipation. It also reduces the power of assimilation in the lower digestive tract.

Nuts and Seeds

Nuts and seeds are very popular in Indian sweet dishes and drinks. They are incorporated into curries and also serve as fillings for *koftas* made of cheese or carrots. Rice dishes can be enriched by the addition of nuts and seeds. Flavored with spices, nuts and seeds are delicious when served with breakfast tea.

Before roasting, nuts must be peeled. Almonds should be soaked overnight before peeling. (Avoid the quicker method of removing the skins by blanching; soaking overnight renders the almonds more digestible.) Nuts can be deep-fried in ghee or vegetable oil until golden brown. Stir constantly while frying to ensure equal browning. After frying, drain the nuts on paper towels and place the nuts in a bowl. Sprinkle with salt, pepper, ground cumin, and ground coriander. Mix well and serve with tea.

Dals

Dried beans, peas, or lentils are referred to collectively as dals. Since dals serve as the main source of protein in an Indian diet, they accompany most meals. There are many ways to cook the same dal; recipes differ from province to province, district to district, city to city, village to village, and house to house. Each family has its own tradition, but they always have something in common. The diversity in cooking styles is due to differences in climate and the chemical nature of the people themselves.

In India, the most popular way to prepare any dal is simply to cook it in water, adding only ground turmeric, ground coriander, and salt. All dals can be prepared this way.

Dals have many uses: they can be prepared as soupy dishes or ground into flour; they can be converted into pastes, to serve as a basis for *koftas, varhis,* or *moongorhis.* They can also be used to fill bread, as with parathas and puris, or simply added to the dough before it is rolled out. Dals can be served plain or with other vegetables added during the cooking. They can be served with different dressings or *tarkas* (spice-flavored ghee), or served with *raitas* (yogurt dishes) or chutneys.

Dals come in many shapes, colors, and sizes, split or whole, with or without skins. Healthy beans are round and have a shine to them. All dals should be cleaned before using. Foreign materials—small stones or sticks—should be removed. To clean, spread the dals on a plate or tray and examine slowly, removing unwanted materials. Most dals must be soaked before cooking (see chart on page 76). When making pastes by hand, soak the dal overnight; if a blender is to be used, 4 to 6 hours will do.

While cooking dals, a foamy residue will collect on top of the water. Remove and discard this scum as it collects.

While urad and moong (mung) beans look very similar except for their skin color, moong beans are easier to digest. All dals, except moong dal, produce gas. People with gallbladder problems might best use skinned dals, as the protein content of the skins contributes to Wind. Soaking and rinsing the dals and using asafoetida or a *dal masala* (spice mixture) while cooking helps to reduce their gaseous effects. A tarka, or spice-flavored ghee (see page 95), added during the preparation of a dal can also help reduce its Wind-producing quality.

It is common practice to remove the children's portions of a dal before adding the tarka, since spicy and hot foods are not suitable for them.

In addition to (or instead of) tarkas, other dressings can be served with dals (see pages 93 and 94): Ghee and cumin seeds, ghee and onions, or ghee and garlic. Since digesting ghee is difficult in the absence of physical exercise, the dressings

DAL	SOAKING TIME	COOKING TIME
Dals are used whole or split, with or without skins.		
Chowla dal		
(black-eyed peas), split	Overnight	1 hour
Chana dal		
(black chick-peas), split	6 hours	1 hour
without skins	6 hours	2 hours
Kabli chana dal		
(garbanzo beans)	Overnight	1½-2 hours
Kala chana dal		
(black chick-peas), whole	Overnight	1-1½ hours
Rajma dal (red kidney beans)	Overnight	1 hour
Moong dal (dried mung beans),		
split/no skins	2 hours	45 minutes
Moong dal		
(dried mung beans), whole	Overnight	1 hour
Moth dal		
(dried dew beans)	2 hours	45 minutes
Masoor dal		
(red lentils), whole	2 hours	1 hour
Masoor dal		
(red lentils), split	2 hours	45 minutes
Matar dal		
(dried split green peas)	Overnight	1½ hours
Toor dal or *arhar dal*		
(yellow lentils)	1-2 hours	1 hour
Urad dal		
(black gram), whole	Overnight	1½ hours
Urad dal		
(black gram), split	1 hour	1 hour

should be used carefully. Healthy, active people can use them over dals or *khichari* (rice and dal combinations) for added taste and to balance their dry natures.

The Spice Mixtures

Since all dals except moong dal produce gases, many recipes include a tarka, a spice-flavored ghee, that makes the dals easy to digest and removes the gas-producing quality.

Masala means any of a number of spice combinations. Sattvic foods* are often cooked with black peppercorns, cardamom (black or green), and cumin. While cumin is a common spice that can be used frequently with rajasic or tamasic foods, it should not be used alone with vegetables that (1) contain a lot of water, (2) are mucus-producing, or (3) are cold in nature. In these cases, it should be used in combination with red chili or black pepper.

Garam masala literally means a "spicy (hot) mixture." It is often used in addition to other spices and/or in recipes that are heavy and oily. Many recipes in this book call for a small amount of a prepared (pre-roasted and ground) garam masala made

---

*See discussion of foods and the three gunas, pages 64–68.

in quantity and kept on hand (see recipe below). A ready-made variety is also available from Indian groceries and some health food stores. Other recipes call for a freshly made garam masala that often is a modified version of the prepared garam masala. The fresh spices in this case are generally not roasted and may be added to the recipe whole or ground. Freshly ground spices lend a more intense flavor than whole spices. Since they do not require cooking,* they are usually added at the end of the cooking process, when the heat is turned off. Some whole spices, such as whole fenugreek seeds or cumin seeds, are added at the beginning of the cooking process. Other whole spices—whole cloves, cardamom, and peppercorns—are often added to soupy dishes that have to cook for a while. These whole spices may also be added near the end of the cooking process to impart a milder flavor and aroma.

Rajasic and tamasic foods can be prepared with garlic, onions, peppers, and fenugreek, or with garam masala. Tamasic foods require more garam masala than do rajasic foods. Ground ginger can be used when vegetables or beans are very gas- or mucus-producing.

All vegetable dishes include a basic masala. One basic masala, made of fenugreek seeds and garlic, sometimes contains cumin seeds and red chili peppers as well. The Basic Soaked Masala, which is called for in many dishes, consists of one part turmeric to two parts ground coriander mixed with water. These two spices are ideal partners, since turmeric is heating and coriander is cooling; in the right proportion (1:2) they balance each other and constitute the basic "curry." In the process of soaking the spices, their water-soluble substances are activated. Sometimes cumin powder, onion, and ginger are added. The soaked masala should have the consistency of thin honey. The container in which the masala was made can be rinsed with 1/4 cup of water and that may be added to the dish being prepared. Since the proportions of soaked masala ingredients vary, the correct amounts are listed in each recipe.

Garam Masala

Yield: 2 1/2 tablespoons

In addition to the spices used in this recipe, garam masala can also include onions, ginger, salt, and green cardamom. Ingredients vary in different parts of India. A small amount of the mixture below, which is called for in many recipes in this book, should be added after the dish has been removed from the heat.

seeds of 1 black cardamom pod
8 whole black peppercorns
4 whole cloves
1 cinnamon stick (2 inches long), broken into small pieces
1/4 teaspoon ground nutmeg
1 teaspoon ground cumin
1 teaspoon ground coriander

Clean and prepare the spices and combine them in a bowl.

In a frying pan, dry-roast half of the spice mixture over low heat until the spices are lightly browned and fragrant. Combine the unroasted spices with the roasted spices and grind in a mortar or electric grinder.

Store the Garam Masala airtight in a glass jar and use whenever called for in a recipe. This mixture will keep for 2 to 3 months without losing its flavor and aroma, but it is best to prepare small amounts and consume within one week.

---

*Turmeric is a spice that should not be eaten uncooked.

The following four masala recipes are for making large quantities to store. Preparing masala in advance can make "fast food" cooking very simple. Small quantities of these masalas can also be taken on trips and to restaurants. It's an easy way to make any meal tastier, more digestible, and healthier. Often these masalas can be found ready made in Indian groceries. They are not fresh, however, as they are shipped from India.

Chat Masala

Yield: 3¼ cups

This masala is to be used in dishes that require a sour taste, such as chutneys or potato fillings for samosas.

> 1 cup cumin seeds
> 2 tablespoons seeds from black cardamom pods
> 4 teaspoons ground cinnamon
> 2 teaspoons ground cloves
> ½ cup ground coriander
> ½ cup whole black peppercorns
> ½ cup mango powder
> ⅓ cup dried pomegranate seeds
> 1½ teaspoons asafoetida powder

Clean and prepare all of the spices; set the mango powder, pomegranate seeds, and asafoetida aside and combine the remaining spices.

In a frying pan, dry-roast half of the combined spice mixture over low heat until the spices are lightly browned and fragrant. Combine the unroasted spices with the roasted spices and grind in a mortar or electric grinder.

Store the Chat Masala airtight in a glass jar and use whenever called for in a recipe. This mixture will keep for 2 to 3 months.

Dal Masala

Yield: 4½ cups

Dal masala is used only with bean or dal dishes. It is an excellent preventative for Wind. Since dals are a main source of protein and form a part of most vegetarian Indian meals, dal masala is a popular, but not required, accompaniment to dal dishes.

> 1 cup ground coriander
> 2 cups cumin seeds
> ¼ cup white salt
> ½ cup whole black peppercorns
> ½ cup black cumin seeds
> 3 tablespoons seeds from black cardamom pods
> ¼ cup black salt
> 2 teaspoons ground cinnamon
> 4 teaspoons ground cloves
> 1 tablespoon asafoetida powder

Clean and prepare all of the spices. Set the asafoetida aside and combine all of the remaining spices.

In a frying pan, dry-roast half of the mixed spices over low heat until the spices are lightly browned and fragrant. Combine the roasted and unroasted spices, and add the asafoetida. Grind the mixture in a mortar or electric grinder to a very fine texture.

Remove the coarse residue with a sieve or strainer and store the Dal Masala airtight in a glass jar. This mixture will keep for 2 to 3 months.

Special Garam Masala #1
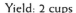
Yield: 2 cups ## with Black Salt and Asafoetida

This masala aids digestion, balances gases, and works as an appetizer. It can be enjoyed by all.

- ½ cup cumin seeds
- ½ cup ground coriander
- ½ cup whole black peppercorns
- 5 teaspoons seeds of black cardamom pods
- 4 teaspoons ground cinnamon
- 2 teaspoons ground cloves
- 2 teaspoons ground nutmeg
- 2 teaspoons black salt
- 1½ teaspoons asafoetida powder

Clean and prepare all of the spices. Set the asafoetida aside and combine all of the remaining spices.

In a frying pan, dry-roast half of the mixed spices over low heat until the spices are lightly browned and fragrant. Combine the roasted and unroasted spices, and add the asafoetida. Grind the mixture in a mortar or electric grinder to a very fine texture.

Remove the coarse residue with a sieve or strainer and store airtight in a glass jar. This mixture will keep for 2 to 3 months.

Special Garam Masala #2

with Ajwain and Saffron

Yield: 2½ cups

This masala is an appetizer. It helps digestion and balances gases, mucus, and heat in the body. To stimulate the appetite, heat 1 teaspoon of this spice mixture in 2 teaspoons of ghee and eat with a piece of bread before a meal. To prevent indigestion, mix ½ teaspoon of this mixture in a glass of warm water and drink it 30 minutes before a meal.

½ cup white cumin seeds
½ cup black cumin seeds
½ cup ground coriander
2½ tablespoons white salt
½ cup ground ginger
5 teaspoons seeds of black cardamom pods
2 teaspoons black salt
½ cup whole black peppercorns
4 teaspoons ground cloves
2½ tablespoons crumbled bay leaves
4 teaspoons ground cinnamon
4 teaspoons fenugreek seeds
4 teaspoons ajwain seeds
2 teaspoons ground nutmeg
2 grams saffron threads, crumbled
2 teaspoons asafoetida powder

Clean and prepare all of the spices. Set the asafoetida aside, and combine all of the remaining spices.

In a frying pan, dry-roast half of the spice mixture over low heat until the spices are lightly browned and fragrant. Combine the roasted and unroasted spices, and add the asafoetida. Grind the mixture in a mortar or electric grinder.

Remove the coarse residue with a sieve or strainer and store airtight in a glass jar. This mixture will keep for 2 to 3 months.

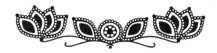

Chapter Two

SNACKS

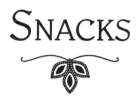

Koftas are deep-fried vegetable or cheese balls.

Paneer Koftas

Serves 4

Basic Paneer (page 178 with all measurements doubled)
¼ cup whole wheat flour, finely sifted
¼ cup filling (dried dal paste, cashew nut paste, or spinach)
8 tablespoons ghee
2 medium onions, chopped
3 cloves garlic, minced
1 teaspoon ground turmeric
2 teaspoons ground coriander
1 cup water
1 medium tomato, quartered
½ teaspoon salt

Mash the paneer and mix with the flour until the texture is spongy. Roll 1 teaspoon of the mixture into a small ball. Flatten it a little and place a small amount of filling in center of each ball. Then roll the ball again.

In a wok, heat 6 tablespoons of the ghee over medium heat. Sauté the balls in batches, turning constantly and adding more ghee as needed, until evenly cooked and golden brown.

In a small bowl, combine the onions, garlic, turmeric, coriander, and water and mash together well.

In a heavy pan, heat the remaining 2 tablespoons ghee. Add the onion mixture and cook until the ghee surfaces. Add the tomato, cooked koftas, and salt and mix well, allowing the flavors to blend.

Serve with Basmati rice or any Indian bread.

Lotus-Root Koftas

Serves 4

2 fresh pieces of lotus root (each about 6 inches), scraped
3 tablespoons chick-pea flour
1 to 2 small fresh green chilis, chopped
1½ teaspoons salt
1 teaspoon Garam Masala (page 77)
8 tablespoons ghee
2 medium onions, chopped
3 cloves garlic, grated
1 teaspoon ground turmeric
2 teaspoons ground coriander
1 cup water
1 medium tomato, quartered

In a heavy pan, cover the lotus roots with water and boil until soft, about 40 to 45 minutes.

Remove from the heat, drain, and add ½ teaspoon of the salt.

In a dry frying pan, roast the chick-pea flour over low heat while stirring. Set aside.

Mash the lotus roots into a fine paste in a mortar or blender. Mix in the chilis, ½ teaspoon salt, Garam Masala, and chick-pea flour. Using one teaspoonful of dough for each, shape the dough into small balls.

In a wok, heat 6 tablespoons of the ghee over medium heat. Sauté the balls in batches, turning constantly, until evenly cooked and golden brown. Remove from the heat and set aside.

In a small bowl, combine the onions, garlic, turmeric, coriander, and water and mash together well.

In a heavy pan, heat the remaining 2 tablespoons ghee. Add the onion mixture and cook until the ghee surfaces. Add the tomato, cooked koftas, and remaining ½ teaspoon salt and mix well, allowing the flavors to blend.

Serve with Basmati rice or any Indian bread.

Carrot-Cashew Koftas

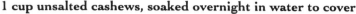

Makes 16, enough to serve 4

1 cup unsalted cashews, soaked overnight in water to cover
¼ teaspoon salt
¾ teaspoon ground cumin
2 cloves garlic, mashed

Basic Soaked Masala:
¼ cup water
1 teaspoon ground turmeric
2 teaspoons ground coriander

½ teaspoon salt
1 teaspoon ground cumin
1 teaspoon Garam Masala (page 77)
3 tablespoons chick-pea flour, dry roasted
4 to 5 medium carrots, finely grated
½ cup ghee or vegetable oil for deep-frying
2 large onions, finely chopped
½ cup plain yogurt
1 medium tomato, quartered
4 small potatoes, peeled and cubed
½ teaspoon salt
hot water

Drain the cashews and mash into a paste in a mortar. Add salt, cumin, and garlic; mix well and set aside.

Combine the basic soaked masala ingredients and let stand for 5 minutes; stir into a thin paste and set aside.

In a bowl, combine the salt, cumin, Garam Masala, and chick-pea flour. Add the carrots and mix to form a nice dough. Pull off chunks of dough and roll into 16 small balls the size of a walnut. Make a hole in the balls with your finger and put a little of the cashew paste into each ball. Seal the balls by rolling between your palms.

Heat the ghee in a wok over medium heat until it is hot but not smoking. Deep fry the balls in batches until golden brown on all sides. Remove the koftas and drain on paper towels.

In the ghee that remains in the wok, sauté the onions until golden brown. Add the soaked masala and cook until the ghee surfaces. Add all of the remaining ingredients, and mix well. Cover and simmer until the potatoes are soft, about 15 to 20 minutes.

Stir in the koftas and add just enough hot water to cover the ingredients. Simmer for a few minutes and remove from the heat. Set aside for the time to allow the flavors to blend.

Serve with a leafy vegetable and puris or chapatis.

Kathal (Jackfruit) Koftas

Serves 4 to 6

$^1/_2$ cup water
$^1/_2$ teaspoon salt
1 pound jackfruit, peeled and cut into $^1/_2$-inch cubes

Masala:
$^1/_2$ teaspoon salt
$^1/_2$ teaspoon ground cinnamon
12 whole black peppercorns
seeds of $1^1/_2$ black cardamom pod
pinch of baking soda

$^1/_2$ cup chick-pea flour
8 tablespoons ghee
2 medium onions, chopped
3 cloves garlic, pressed or minced
1 teaspoon ground turmeric
2 teaspoons ground coriander
1 cup water
1 medium tomato, quartered
$^1/_2$ teaspoon salt

Place water and salt in a heavy pan, and steam the jackfruit until soft, about 30 to 35 minutes. Remove from the heat and drain. Mash the jackfruit into a fine paste in a mortar or blender.

Grind all of the masala ingredients into a fine powder and add to the jackfruit mixture.

In a dry frying pan, roast the chick-pea flour over low heat while stirring. Add the flour to the jackfruit mixture and stir to make a dough that is dry enough to roll into small (walnut-size) balls, yet moist enough not to crumble.

Heat 6 tablespoons of the ghee in a wok over medium heat. Sauté the balls, turning constantly, until evenly cooked. Remove and set aside.

In a small bowl, combine the onions, garlic, turmeric, coriander, and water and mash together well.

In a heavy pan, heat the remaining 2 tablespoons ghee. Add the onion mixture and cook until the ghee surfaces. Add the tomato, cooked koftas, and salt, and mix well, allowing the flavors to blend. For a thinner, soupier dish, add 1 cup of hot water and simmer over low heat.

Serve with chapatis or puris and a vegetable dish.

Dry Yam-Potato-Cashew Koftas

Serves 6 to 8

    1 large Indian yam (suran)
    2 large potatoes

Garam Masala (finely ground):
    8 whole cloves
    8 whole black peppercorns
    1 medium onion, finely grated
    1 teaspoon ground ginger
    ¹/₂ cup fresh coriander leaves, whole

    1 cup unsalted cashews, soaked in water to cover for 8 to 10 hours
    1 teaspoon salt
    1 cup chick-pea flour, roasted and sifted

Basic Soaked Masala:
    ¹/₂ cup water
    1 teaspoon ground turmeric
    2 teaspoons ground coriander

    2 tablespoons ghee
    2 large onions, finely chopped

Preheat the oven to 400 degrees F.

Puncture the yams and potatoes with a fork and bake for 1 hour. (They can also be cooked over an open fire or boiled until soft.) Peel the yams and potatoes and mash together in a large bowl; set aside. Prepare the garam masala.

Grind the cashews into a fine paste in a blender or mortar. Add the salt and 1 teaspoon of the garam masala to the cashews. Add the chick-pea flour and mix well. Using 1 teaspoonful of the mixture, form a patty 1-inch in diameter and ¹/₂ inch thick. Add more chick-pea flour if the mixture is too loose. Continue to shape the patties (24 to 32) until no more paste remains; set aside.

Combine the basic soaked masala ingredients and let stand for 5 minutes; stir into a thin paste.

In a heavy pan, heat the ghee over medium heat. Add the onions and cook until golden brown and the ghee surfaces. Stir in the soaked masala and cook until the ghee surfaces again. Drop the koftas into the mixture, cover, and cook for 30–40 minutes, until the ghee surfaces. Add water and salt as needed.

Serve with chapatis or parathas.

Samosas are vegetable-filled pastries often eaten as snacks with tea.

Fried-Potato Samosas

Makes 14

Filling:
  1 tablespoon ghee, for frying
  2 medium potatoes, peeled and coarsely grated
  1 teaspoon dried pomegranate seeds, finely ground
  ½ teaspoon Dal Masala (page 78)
  ½ teaspoon oregano seeds
  ¼ teaspoon mango powder
  ¼ teaspoon fenugreek seeds
  ¼ teaspoon salt

Dough:
  1½ cups finely ground whole wheat flour
  2 tablespoons ghee
  1 teaspoon oregano seeds
  ½ teaspoon salt
  about ⅓ cup water
  5 tablespoons ghee, for frying samosas

In a frying pan, warm 1 tablespoon ghee over medium-low heat. Add the potatoes and all of the other filling ingredients and cook until tender, about 30 minutes.

To make the samosa dough, combine the flour, 2 tablespoons ghee, oregano seeds, and salt. Add slightly less than ⅓ cup of water and knead until elastic, firm, and non-sticky. Pinch off walnut-size balls of dough and roll each into a thin 4-inch patty. Cut each patty in half and wet half of straight edge of each half-circle with a few drops of water. Fold one corner over the other, wet edge first, to form a funnel-shaped pouch. Firmly seal the edges and fill the pouch two-thirds full with the potato mixture. With moist fingertips, wet the inside of the top opening and pinch closed. Repeat until all of the samosas are formed.

In a frying pan, heat the 5 tablespoons ghee over medium-low heat. When ghee is hot but not smoking, fry the samosas in small batches until golden brown on all sides, about 5 to 8 minutes. Drain on paper towels. Serve with a saunth or chutney (or natural ketchup).

Snacks

Boiled-Potato Samosas

Makes 24

Filling:
 6 medium potatoes, boiled and peeled
 1 teaspoon mango powder
 1 teaspoon dried pomegranate seeds, finely ground
 1 teaspoon Dal Masala (page 78)
 $^1/_2$ teaspoon oregano seeds
 $^1/_2$ teaspoon ground ginger, or 2 teaspoons chopped fresh ginger
 1 teaspoon salt
 1 to 2 cups shelled fresh green peas, cooked (optional)
 1 cup ghee (for frying)

In a bowl, break the boiled potatoes into small pieces and combine with all of the remaining filling ingredients. Mix well.

Make the samosa dough and pouches according to the preceding recipe. Fill pouches with the potato mixture. Fry two samosas at a time in the ghee over medium-low heat until browned on all sides, about 5 to 6 minutes. Serve with a saunth or chutney.

Variation

Sauté the potato mixture in ghee before filling the samosa pouches. (Some may find this makes the dish difficult to digest, but children and young people will have no difficulty digesting it.)

Potato Kachoris

Makes 4

Kachoris are deep-fried savories eaten for breakfast, as a snack, or with a main meal. In North Indian feasts, they are made by expert cooks who shape the dough by hand without using a rolling pin.

Dough:
$^{1}/_{2}$ cup whole wheat or chapati flour
$^{1}/_{8}$ teaspoon salt
$^{1}/_{4}$ teaspoon oregano seeds
$^{1}/_{4}$ teaspoon asafoetida powder
6 tablespoons water

Filling:
2 small potatoes, boiled, peeled, and mashed
$^{1}/_{8}$ teaspoon salt
$^{1}/_{4}$ teaspoon ground cumin
$^{1}/_{2}$ teaspoon coarsely ground fennel or anise seeds
$^{1}/_{4}$ teaspoon ground coriander
$^{1}/_{4}$ teaspoon ground ginger
$^{1}/_{4}$ teaspoon Garam Masala (page 77)
1 cup ghee or vegetable oil for deep-frying

To prepare the dough, sift flour into a deep bowl; add the salt and oregano seeds. In a small bowl, dissolve the asafoetida in the water. Make a hole in the middle of the dry ingredients and add the liquid. Mix well by hand until a smooth ball forms. Add more flour or water as needed to achieve a workable, elastic consistency; the dough should not stick to the fingers or be dry or hard. With your knuckles, make a few indentations in the dough and sprinkle with a little water. Cover with an inverted bowl or clean kitchen towel and allow to stand for 30 minutes. Kachori dough should be softer than puri, paratha, or chapati dough.

To prepare the filling, combine the potatoes with the salt and spices and mix well.

To make the kachoris, knead the dough once more before using, if time permits. Divide the dough into 4 plum-size balls. Place a drop of ghee on one hand and roll one ball between your palms. Flatten the ball into a 2-inch-diameter patty about $^{1}/_{8}$ inch thick. Make a depression in the center with your finger and stuff with 1 teaspoon of the filling. Fold the sides of the dough over the filling and pinch the seams together on all sides. Roll the ball gently between the palms, without applying pressure. Sprinkle a few drops of ghee on a rolling board and roll ball gently into a patty about $3^{1}/_{2}$ inches in diameter. The edges should be slightly thinner than the center.

Deep-fry according to the puris recipe (page 214).

Mixed-Vegetable Pakora

Serves 4 to 6

Pakoras are batter-coated deep-fried vegetables often served as a snack with chutney or saunth, and lemon juice or vinegar. They increase acidity and should be eaten in moderation. (Because they are very tasty, it is always tempting to eat too many.)

    2 cups chick-pea flour
    1½ cups water
    1 teaspoon ground turmeric
    1 teaspoon ground coriander
    1 teaspoon ground cumin
    1 teaspoon oregano seeds
    ½ teaspoon salt
    1 teaspoon ground ginger
    pinch of ground cinnamon
    ¼ teaspoon asafoetida powder
    1 teaspoon crushed dried fenugreek (*methi*) leaves (optional), soaked*
    ½ cup ghee or vegetable oil for shallow-frying

    1 eggplant, peeled and thinly sliced
    4 medium potatoes, peeled and thinly sliced
    1 green bell pepper, thinly sliced
    2 tablespoons fresh mushrooms, thinly sliced
    2 tablespoons coarsely chopped fresh spinach

Sift the chick-pea flour into a bowl and add the water, a little at a time, until a paste forms. Add all of the spices and whip the paste with an egg beater or in a blender. Drop a small amount of the mixture into a cup of water. If the paste floats, it is ready to cook.

In a heavy pan or wok, heat the ghee over medium heat. When the ghee is hot but not smoking, dip the vegetables, one piece at a time, into the chickpea paste (make sure vegetables are completely covered by the paste) and place into the hot ghee. Stir constantly until well cooked and golden brown. Remove with a slotted spoon and drain the pakora on paper towels. Continue dipping and frying until all the vegetables are cooked.

Serve with vinegar pickle, lemon, chutney, or saunth.

*Note: Dried fenugreek leaves should be soaked in water for 5 minutes and then stirred with the fingertips. The dust that settles to the bottom is not good to digest and should be discarded.

The recipes that follow are for salty snacks to serve between meals
or with tea in the afternoon or evening.

Vegetable Chips

Serves 4

½ cup ghee or vegetable oil
1 cup thinly sliced mixed vegetables, such as potatoes, carrots,
    plantains, and eggplant, patted dry
1 teaspoon ground cumin
1 teaspoon ground coriander
pinch of mango powder
salt and pepper, to taste

In a wok, heat the ghee over medium heat. Drop in vegetable slices and cook, stirring constantly, until crisp and slightly brown. Drain on paper towels.

Meanwhile, combine the remaining ingredients.

Sprinkle the chips with the spice mixture (or 2 teaspoons Garam Masala, page 77).

Eggplant Chips

Serves 4

Vegetable oil or ghee for deep-frying
1 large eggplant, washed and thinly sliced

Masala:
    1 teaspoon salt
    ½ teaspoon black peppercorns (freshly ground)
    1 teaspoon ground coriander
    1 teaspoon ground cumin

In a wok, heat the oil over medium heat until hot but not smoking. Fry the eggplant slices in batches until crisp. Remove from the heat.

Sprinkle the eggplant chips with the masala and serve as a snack or with a meal. Chips from potatoes or green bananas (plantains) can also be prepared in this way.

Buckwheat Pakoras

Serves 4

Batter:
> 1 cup buckwheat flour
> ¹/₂ teaspoon ground ginger
> pinch of asafoetida powder
> 1 tablespoon dried fenugreek (*methi*) leaves, soaked*
> ¹/₂ teaspoon salt
> 2 tablespoons water
>
> ¹/₂ to 1 cup vegetable pieces, such as potatoes, onion rings, spinach, or
> plantain slices
> ¹/₂ cup ghee or vegetable oil

To make the batter, combine all of the batter ingredients in a shallow bowl and mix well to form a thick paste. Drop the vegetable pieces into the paste and turn to coat well.

In a deep wok, heat the ghee over medium heat. Add the battered vegetables, one at a time, and deep-fry, stirring constantly, until well cooked and crisp.

Serve with raita, salad, chutney, or saunth, or vinegar or ginger pickle

Variation

> Precooked vegetables, such as leftover beans, cauliflower, or cumin potatoes, can be used here. Make a simple paste from flour, ground ginger, and water (some salt and spices will already be present from first cooking).

*Note: Dried fenugreek leaves should be soaked in water for 5 minutes and then stirred with the fingertips. The dust that settles to the bottom is not good to digest and should be discarded.

*The following recipes are for roasted seeds and nuts, which are
especially nourishing when taken together with raisins.*

Roasted Sunflower Seeds

Serves 2

¹/₄ to ¹/₃ cup unsalted sunflower seeds
¹/₄ teaspoon ghee

Masala:
¹/₂ teaspoon ground cumin
³/₄ teaspoon ground coriander
¹/₈ teaspoon salt
¹/₈ teaspoon freshly ground black pepper
pinch of black salt

In a dry frying pan over a low heat, dry-roast the seeds. Stir constantly to
ensure even browning. Remove to a bowl and add the ghee. Sprinkle with
the masala and mix well. Serve with tea.

Variation

Honeydew melon and cantaloupe seeds can also be prepared in this way.

Roasted Cashews with Masala

Serves 4

1 cup unsalted cashews
¹/₄ teaspoon ghee

Masala:
¹/₄ teaspoon salt
¹/₂ teaspoon freshly ground black pepper
1 teaspoon ground coriander
1 teaspoon ground cumin
pinch of mango powder
pinch of black salt

Preheat a wok or heavy pan over medium-low heat. Dry-roast cashews until
they turn golden brown. Remove the nuts to a bowl and sprinkle with the
ghee and masala ingredients; mix well.

Serve with tea.

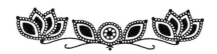

Chapter Three

DALS

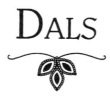

DRESSINGS FOR DAL DISHES

Onion Dressing
---

1 teaspoon ghee (per person)
¹/₂ medium onion (per person), chopped

Heat the ghee in a small frying pan. Add the onion and sauté until golden brown and the ghee surfaces again. Remove from the heat.

Note: When cooking for one person, 1 tablespoon of ghee should be used to prevent the onion or garlic from burning.

Garlic Dressing
---

1 teaspoon ghee (per person)
¹/₂ to 1 clove garlic (per person), finely sliced

Heat the ghee in a small frying pan. Add the garlic and sauté until golden brown and the ghee surfaces again. Remove from the heat.

Note: When cooking for one person, 1 tablespoon of ghee should be used to prevent the onion or garlic from burning.

Onion-Garlic Dressing

Serves 4

4 teaspoons ghee
1 to 2 medium onions, chopped
2 cloves garlic, finely sliced

Heat the ghee in a small frying pan. Add the garlic and sauté until golden brown, then add the onion and sauté until it is golden brown and the ghee surfaces again. Remove from the heat.

Cumin Seed Dressing

Serves 4

¼ cup ghee
½ teaspoon cumin seeds

Heat the ghee in a small frying pan. Add the cumin seeds and sauté until golden brown. Remove from the heat.

TARKAS

A tarka, or spice-flavored ghee, is prepared and added to a dish just before serving. There are two popular types of tarkas: those made with garlic and dried red pepper, and those made with cumin, cardamom, and cloves. Both contain a pinch of asafoetida powder. This book contains these tarkas, as well as variations on them. With moong dal, the cumin seed tarka is usually used.

Basic Tarka

Serves 4

  1 tablespoon ghee
  1 teaspoon minced garlic
  1 dried red chili (crushed or whole)
  ½ teaspoon asafoetida powder
  1 teaspoon cumin seeds

In a ladle or small frying pan, heat the ghee. Add the spices and sauté for a few minutes, until well-toasted and fragrant. Add the tarka to the dal dish and cover immediately with a tight-fitting lid. Allow to stand for a few minutes while the flavors blend.

Variation

  When making a moong bean dal, use the seeds of 1 black cardamom pod, 2 whole cloves, and 1 teaspoon black cumin seeds.

DAL DISHES

A Basic Dal Dish

Serves 4

  4 cups cold water
  1 teaspoon ground turmeric
  2 teaspoons ground coriander
  1 cup any dal (dried beans, peas, or lentils), washed, soaked, and drained
  1 teaspoon salt
  Basic Tarka (recipe above)

In a heavy saucepan, bring the water to a boil. Add the spices, dal, and salt. Cover, and cook over medium heat for 45 minutes, or until the dal is soft and can be mashed easily with a spoon. Remove from the heat and allow to cool for about 20 minutes.

  Add the Tarka and drizzle with lemon juice or top with thin slices of ginger pickled in lemon to aid digestion.

ABOUT MOONG DAL

Dried moong (mung) beans are available with or without skins. With skins, they are light, provide roughage for the digestive system, and can be eaten by people of all ages. They are also available whole or split. Split moong (mung) beans, which are very popular in North India, are often served to people with weak stomachs.

Healthy people eat moong dal for its protein value. It is especially good for children and those who are weak or ill. Moong beans are good for people interested in spiritual work as well as those who wish to enjoy a healthy sexual life. They increase virility and provide physical strength. There is a saying in Hindi about moong dal:

> *Ya khaye rogi, Ya khaye yogi, Yo khaye bhogi.*
> Either sick people eat it, or Yogis eat it,
> or Bhogis [people who enjoy sensual pleasures] eat it.

Split Moong Dal and Spinach

Serves 4

4 cups water
1 teaspoon ground turmeric
2 teaspoons ground coriander
1 cup split and peeled moong dal, washed, soaked, and drained
6 to 8 ounces fresh spinach, washed well and stemmed

Tarka:
1 tablespoon ghee
3/4 teaspoon black cumin seeds
seeds of 1 black cardamom pod
4 whole cloves
pinch of asafoetida powder

In a cast-iron pot, boil the water with the ground turmeric and coriander. Add the moong beans, cover, and boil for 10 to 15 minutes. Stir in the spinach, cover, and simmer over medium-low heat for 30 to 35 minutes, or until moong beans can be easily mashed. Remove from the heat.

To make the tarka, heat the ghee in a ladle or small frying pan. Add the spices and sauté until well-toasted and fragrant.

Add the sizzling tarka to the dal and immediately cover the pot with a tight-fitting lid. Allow to stand for a few minutes, while the flavors blend.

Serve with chapatis, puris, pickled ginger, and a vegetable dish.

Split Moong Dal with Masala

Serves 4

    4 cups water
    ¹/₄ teaspoon ground turmeric
    ¹/₂ teaspoon ground coriander
    ¹/₂ teaspoon salt
    1 cup split and peeled moong beans, washed, soaked, and drained

Masala:
    seeds of 1 black cardamom pod
    4 whole cloves
    4 to 6 bay leaves, crumbled
    8 black peppercorns
    pinch of saffron

Tarka:
    1 tablespoon ghee
    1 teaspoon black cumin seeds

In a heavy saucepan, bring the water to a boil, and add the turmeric, coriander, and salt. Add the moong beans, cover, and cook over medium heat for 45 minutes, or until the dal is soft and can easily be mashed with a spoon.

Add the remaining ingredients, except the tarka, and simmer over low heat for 5 minutes. Remove from the heat.

To prepare the tarka, heat the ghee in a ladle or small frying pan. Add the cumin seeds and sauté until well-toasted and fragrant.

Add the tarka to the dal and cover immediately with a tight-fitting lid. Allow to stand for a few minutes, while the flavors blend. Serve with rice and any Indian bread.

Eggplant with Moong Beans

Serves 4

1 large eggplant

Soaked Masala:
  $\frac{1}{2}$ cup water
  1 teaspoon ground turmeric
  2 teaspoons ground coriander
  1 teaspoon ground cumin

1 cup split and peeled moong beans, washed, soaked, and drained
3 cups water
$1\frac{1}{2}$ teaspoons salt
2 tablespoons ghee
2 cloves garlic, chopped
1 teaspoon fenugreek seeds
$\frac{1}{2}$ to 1 dried red chili pepper, crushed (optional)
2 medium onions, chopped
1 large tomato, quartered
$\frac{1}{2}$ teaspoon ground cinnamon

Preheat the oven to 400 degrees F.

Wash the eggplant and pierce in several places with a fork. Place the eggplant in a pan and bake for 45 minutes, or until soft.

Meanwhile, prepare the soaked masala by soaking the spices in the water for 5 minutes; stir into a thin paste and set aside.

In a heavy saucepan, heat the water and $\frac{1}{2}$ teaspoon of the salt. Add the beans, cover, and cook over medium heat for 45 minutes, or until the beans become soft and the liquid is absorbed.

In a wok, heat the ghee. Add the garlic and sauté until light brown. Add the fenugreek seeds, chili pepper, and onion and sauté until the ghee surfaces. Stir in the soaked masala and continue cooking until the ghee surfaces again. Add the tomato and cook until dissolved.

When the eggplant is cool enough to handle, peel it and mash the pulpy interior.

In a heavy saucepan, combine the eggplant pulp and the sautéed spice mixture, stirring well. Add the cooked moong beans and the remaining 1 teaspoon salt. Mix well and simmer over low heat for 10 minutes.

Stir in the cinnamon and allow the flavors to blend for a few minutes.

Serve with any Indian bread and saunth.

Split Moong Beans with Cumin

Serves 4

This makes an ideal breakfast dish.

> **2 tablespoons ghee**
> **1 tablespoon black cumin seeds**
> **1 dried red chili pepper, crushed**
> **pinch of asafoetida powder**
> **1 cup split and peeled moong beans, washed, soaked, and drained**
> **1 teaspoon salt**
> **2 cups water**
> **1 teaspoon ground cumin**
> **juice of 1 lemon**

In a wok, heat the ghee over medium heat. Add the cumin seeds, chili pepper, and asafoetida and sauté until the cumin turns light brown. Mix in the moong beans and salt and sauté, stirring constantly, for 10 minutes.

Reduce the heat, add the water, and cook over medium-low heat for 35 minutes, or until the beans are soft and the water evaporates. Stir in the ground cumin and cover.

To serve, drizzle with the lemon juice and accompany with your favorite Indian bread.

Black Chick-peas with Ajwain

Serves 4

> **1 tablespoon ghee**
> **1 tablespoon ajwain seeds**
> **1 dried red chili pepper, crushed**
> **pinch of asafoetida powder**
> **1 cup whole black chick-peas (*kala chana*), washed, soaked for 24 to 36 hours, and drained**
> **1 teaspoon salt**
> **1 teaspoon baking soda**
> **water to cover, for cooking**

In a heavy saucepan, heat the ghee over medium heat. Add the ajwain seeds, chili pepper, and asafoetida. Mix in the chick-peas, salt, baking soda, and enough water to cover. Cover and cook over medium heat for 1 to 1½ hours, or until the beans are soft and the water is absorbed.

Serve with puris and ginger pickles.

Split Moong Dal with Ghee

Serves 4

1 cup split and peeled moong beans, washed and soaked for 1 hour in
   4 cups of water
1/2 cup ghee

Masala:
   1 teaspoon black cumin seeds
   2 whole black peppercorns
   1/2 teaspoon ground coriander
   1/4 teaspoon ground turmeric
   6 to 8 bay leaves, crumbled
   1 teaspoon salt

Tarka:
   1 teaspoon ghee
   1/2 teaspoon black cumin seeds
   1 garlic clove, crushed
   pinch of asafoetida powder

Drain the moong beans and reserve the soaking water.

In a heavy saucepan, bring the soaking water to a boil. Add the beans,
cover, and simmer over medium heat for 45 minutes, or until soft.

In a large, heavy pan, heat 1/4 cup of the ghee. Add all of the masala ingredients and cook until fragrant and the ghee surfaces. Stir in the cooked
moong beans and their cooking water, and the salt. Cover and bring the mixture to a gentle boil. Continue to cook, covered, over medium heat for 10 to
15 minutes, or until the beans are soft and the liquid is absorbed.

Stir in the remaining 1/4 cup ghee and cover the pan.

To prepare the tarka, heat the ghee in a ladle or small frying pan. Add
the tarka spices and sauté until well-toasted and fragrant. Add the sizzling
tarka to the dal and cover immediately with a tight-fitting lid. Allow to stand
for a few minutes, while the flavors blend. Stir and remove the spoon.

Serve with rice and an Indian bread.

Variation
   Zucchini, tomato, fresh fenugreek leaves, or spinach can
   be added to the dal, but these vegetables must always be
   accompanied by a sour-tasting spice, such as pomegranate
   seeds or mango powder.

Moongorhi and Varhi with Rice

Serves 2

Moongorhis are dumplings made with moong dal paste, black pepper, cumin, and salt. Varhis, or badis, are dumplings made with urad dal and Chinese squash. All these dumplings are sun-dried and sold in Indian groceries.

> **2 cups Basmati rice, cleaned and soaked for 2 to 3 hours**
> **2 tablespoons ghee**
> **½ cup (or handful) moongorhi balls**
> **2 pieces varhi (each the size of a lime)**
> **1 teaspoon black cumin seeds**
> **1 dried red chili pepper, crushed (optional)**
> **¼ teaspoon asafoetida powder**
> **2 medium onions, finely chopped**
> **4 cups water**
> **1 teaspoon salt**

Garam Masala (whole, optional):
> **2 whole cloves**
> **4 whole black peppercorns**
> **seeds of ½ black cardamom pod, ground**
> **2 bay leaves**
> **1 cinnamon stick (2 inches long)**

Drain the rice and discard the soaking water. In a wok, heat the ghee over medium-low heat. Add the moongorhis and varhi and sauté until light brown on all sides. Remove from the wok and set aside.

Add the cumin seeds, chili pepper, and asafoetida to the wok. Sauté until the seeds pop. Add the onions and sauté until light brown and the ghee surfaces. Stirring constantly, add the rice and sauté for 2 minutes. Add the moongorhis and varhi, the water, and salt. Cover and bring to a boil. Garam Masala may be added, if desired. Simmer until the rice is cooked, 35 to 40 minutes.

Meanwhile, preheat the oven to 450 degrees F.

Place the wok, tightly covered, in the oven and turn off the heat. Allow to sit 5 to 10 minutes to remove excess moisture.

Serve with raita and pappadams or with saunth or fresh chutney.

Bean Balls in Yogurt (Dahi Balla)

Serves 8

Dahi Balla are fried dal balls.

2 cups split and peeled urad beans, soaked overnight in water to cover
1 teaspoon salt
1½ teaspoons Dal Masala (page 78)
6 tablespoons ghee
bowl of hot water
1 cup plain yogurt
pinch of salt
pinch of pepper

Tarka:
1 tablespoon ghee
½ teaspoon black cumin seeds
1 teaspoon sesame seeds
pinch of asafoetida powder

Drain the soaked beans and pat dry with a clean kitchen towel. Grind the beans to a fine paste in a mortar or blender. The paste should be very dry. Add the salt to the Dal Masala. In a bowl, combine the bean paste and Dal Masala mixture. Form into 16 small balls and set aside.

In a wok, heat the ghee over medium heat. Working in batches, place several balls into the hot ghee and deep-fry until golden brown on all sides. Remove the cooked balls to a bowl of hot water and soak for 30 minutes to 1 hour, until the oil exudes. Remove and gently squeeze out any excess water.

In a bowl, combine the yogurt, salt, and pepper; cover and set aside.

To prepare the tarka, heat the ghee in a ladle or small frying pan. Add the cumin and sesame seeds and sauté until well-toasted and fragrant. Add the asafoetida and pour the sizzling tarka into the bowl of yogurt. Cover immediately and let stand for 5 minutes. Stir the tarka into the yogurt and add the bean balls.

Serve with puris or chapatis and saunth.

Variations

Place the bean balls on a clean, wet cloth and press into thin ⅛- to ¼-inch thick patties. Cut out 2-inch circles of dough. Follow the cooking method given in recipe.

For a sweeter treat, soak the following in water to cover: 1 cup raisins, for 30 to 60 minutes; 1 cup of mixed nuts (almonds, cashews, and pistachios) for 4 hours. Peel the almonds; finely chop all nuts, and combine with raisins. If desired, add 2 tablespoons grated dried coconut or coconut powder. Place ½ teaspoon of this mixture on an uncooked patty. Cover with a second patty and seal the edges firmly with fingertips. Follow the instructions given in the recipe for cooking the bean balls and making the tarka.

Mixed Dal Stew with Tarka

Serves 4

> 1 cup dal (equal parts of split toor, moong, urad; whole or split black chick-peas [peeled or with skins]; peeled red lentils), soaked separately (see chart, page 76)
> 4 cups water
> 1 teaspoon ground turmeric
> 2 teaspoons ground coriander
> 1 teaspoon salt
> 1 teaspoon mango powder or finely crushed dried pomegranate seeds

Tarka:
> 1 tablespoon ghee
> 2 cloves garlic, crushed
> 1/8 teaspoon black cumin seeds
> 1 small dried red chili pepper, crushed
> pinch of asafoetida powder
> Onion Dressing (page 93)
> Dal Masala (page 78) (optional)

Drain the dals and discard the soaking water.

In a heavy saucepan, bring the 4 cups water, turmeric, coriander, and salt to a boil. Stir in the drained dals, cover, and simmer over medium heat for 1 to 1 1/2 hours, or until soft. Remove from the heat and stir in the mango powder.

To prepare the tarka, heat the ghee in a ladle or small frying pan. Add the tarka ingredients and sauté until well-toasted and fragrant. Add the sizzling tarka to the dal and cover immediately. Allow to stand for a few minutes, while the flavors blend. Just before serving, pour 1 teaspoonful of the Onion Dressing atop each bowl of stew. Dal Masala can also be sprinkled over individual servings if a spicy taste is desired.

Rice and Urad Dal Pancakes (Chila)

Serves 4

This recipe will make 10 to 15 pancakes, each 5¹/₂ inches in diameter.

> ¹/₂ cup Basmati rice, soaked overnight
> ¹/₂ cup split and peeled urad dal, soaked overnight
> 1 teaspoon salt
> 1 teaspoon Garam Masala (page 77)
> 1 teaspoon mango powder
> 1 teaspoon ground cumin
> pinch of asafoetida powder
> about ¹/₃ cup ghee

Drain the rice and dal and grind the mixture in a mortar to a thin paste. Add the salt and spices and mix well.

In a nonstick frying pan, heat 1 teaspoon of the ghee over medium-low heat. Ladle in a small amount of the thin, spiced batter and tilt the pan to coat the bottom. Cook until the pancake turns golden brown. Add more ghee with each pancake and continue until no batter remains.

Serve with chutney or saunth.

Lentil Kababs

Serves 6

Kababs are small balls (one inch in diameter) made with dal paste that has been dried over low heat. Kababs can be used dry or in soup.

**1 cup red lentils (*masoor dal*), washed and soaked overnight, and
  drained**
3 tablespoons ghee, plus additional for shallow-frying
1 teaspoon salt
1 teaspoon Garam Masala (page 77)

Basic Soaked Masala:
  ¹/₂ cup water
  1 teaspoon ground turmeric
  2 teaspoons ground coriander

  1 teaspoon fenugreek seeds
  3 garlic cloves, sliced
  6 medium onions, chopped
  1 medium tomato, quartered
  1 teaspoon salt
  1 medium red beet, grated
  12 whole black peppercorns
  seeds of 1¹/₂ black cardamom pods
  1 teaspoon ground ginger
  1 whole clove
  pinch of ground cinnamon

Grind the drained lentils in a mortar. Whip the mixture into a paste with an egg beater. (A blender can be used to combine these two steps.)

Heat 1 tablespoon of the ghee over medium heat in a heavy pan or wok. When the ghee is hot but not smoking, drop in the entire paste mixture. Stir with a spatula and cook over low heat until the mixture thickens and changes color, about 20 to 25 minutes. Turn off the heat and stir in the salt and Garam Masala. Allow the lentil paste to cool.

Roll the paste into 1-inch balls.

In a heavy pan or wok, heat enough ghee for shallow-frying. When the ghee is hot, fry the balls, turning carefully, until golden brown.

Combine the ingredients for the basic soaked masala and set aside for 5 minutes.

In a large heavy pan, heat the remaining 2 tablespoons ghee and add the fenugreek seeds, garlic, half of the onions, and the tomato. Sauté for a few minutes, and add the soaked masala, salt, beet, and the remaining onions. When the beet softens, add the fried balls and cover. Cook for 20 minutes. Add all of the remaining ingredients and cook for another 5 minutes.

Serve with parathas or rice.

Katra with Red Lentils

Katra are ¹/₂-inch cubes of fried lentil paste.

  1 cup red lentils (*masoor dal*), washed, soaked overnight, and drained
  1 teaspoon Garam Masala (page 77)
  3 tablespoons ghee, plus additional for shallow-frying

Basic Soaked Masala:
  ¹/₂ cup water
  1 teaspoon ground turmeric
  2 teaspoons ground coriander

  1 teaspoon fenugreek seeds
  2 large onions, chopped
  1 medium tomato, quartered
  2 green chicories (Belgian endive), sliced in rounds
  1 teaspoon salt
  seeds of 1 red cardamom pod
  8 whole black peppercorns
  4 whole cloves
  1 teaspoon salt
  ¹/₂ teaspoon ground ginger
  ¹/₄ teaspoon ground cinnamon

Grind the drained lentils in a mortar. Whip the mixture into a paste with an egg beater. (A blender can be used to combine these two steps.)

In a heavy pan or wok, heat 1 tablespoon of the ghee over medium heat. When the ghee is hot but not smoking, drop in the paste mixture. Cook over low heat to remove remaining moisture. Stir with a spatula until the mixture thickens and changes color, about 20–25 minutes. Add the Garam Masala. When the paste is dry, remove from the heat and place on a cutting board to cool.

Roll out the paste about ¹/₂ inch thick and cut into ¹/₂-inch cubes.

In a wok, heat enough ghee for shallow-frying and fry the lentil cubes, turning carefully, until brown. Remove from the wok and set aside.

Combine the basic soaked masala ingredients and let stand for 5 minutes; stir into a thin paste and set aside.

Heat the remaining 2 tablespoons ghee in the wok. Add the fenugreek seeds and onions and sauté until the onions change color. Add the soaked masala and cook until the ghee surfaces. Add the tomato and cook until it dissolves into the other ingredients. Add the chicories and the salt (and a little water if needed), and cook over low heat until the ghee surfaces again. Add the lentil cubes and simmer a few minutes more.

Remove from heat and add all of the remaining ingredients. Allow the flavors to blend.

Serve with chapatis, puris, or parathas.

DAL SOUPS (OR SOUPY DISHES)

Soups in an Indian kitchen are different from Western soups, which are served before the main meal as an appetizer. Indian soups are served with the main meal to complement and soften the customary boiled rice or fresh, unleavened breads. While Western soups frequently contain cornstarch or other thickeners, Indian soups are naturally thick, closer to the consistency of stew. They are usually made from dal and/or vegetables with spices. Sometimes a special soup is made from buttermilk or liquefied yogurt, known as *kadhi*. In southern Indian cooking a soup made from a mixture of dal and vegetables is served with a stuffed bread known as *dosa*. Curried soups made from vegetables, paneer, dal, or a combination of dal and vegetables are served throughout India. Their purpose is to excite the taste buds, enhance the digestive juices, and add flavor to unsalted breads or rice. A typical Indian lunch or dinner consists of rice and/or bread, a dry vegetable or dal dish, and a soupy curry.

Arwi Root (Taro) Soup

Serves 4

mustard oil (enough to coat hands)
6 to 8 medium arwi roots (taro)
3 tablespoons mustard (or other vegetable) oil or ghee
4 to 6 cloves garlic, chopped
1 dried red chili pepper, crushed
6 medium onions (or weight equivalent to arwi)
1 teaspoon fenugreek seeds
¹/₄ cup water
1 teaspoon salt

Apply a small amount of mustard oil or ghee (other oils are not as effective) to hands to avoid a tingling sensation in the fingertips from handling the arwi root. Peel the arwi with a knife and cut it into ¹/₂-inch cubes.

In a medium saucepan, heat the oil over medium heat. Add the garlic and sauté until brown. Add the following ingredients in order: the chili pepper, onions, fenugreek seeds, arwi root, water, and salt. Cover and simmer over medium heat for about 35 minutes, or until arwi root is soft. Allow flavors to blend.

Serve with any kind of Indian bread—puris, chapatis, or parathas.

Buttermilk Soup (Kadhi)

with Chick-pea Flour
Serves 8

This dish has a golden yellow color and is spicy as well as sour. It is good for curing stomach disorders or soothing an upset digestive system. The buttermilk should not be too sour, however, or the dish will not be soothing and will create acidity.

> 1 cup chick-pea flour
> 1/2 cup water
> 1 teaspoon ground turmeric
> 1 teaspoon salt
> 6 cups buttermilk
> 6 tablespoons ghee
> 1 teaspoon fenugreek seeds
> 2 dried red chili peppers, crushed
> 1/4 teaspoon asafoetida powder

Topping:
> 3 tablespoons ghee
> 1 teaspoon coriander seeds

Soak the chick-pea flour in the 1/2 cup of water for 5 minutes. Add the turmeric and salt and stir into a thin paste. Whip with an egg beater, as if whipping cream. Test the paste by dropping a small amount of it into a cup of warm water. When the paste has been whipped enough, it floats and is ready to cook.

Mix one-fourth of the chick-pea paste with 2 cups of the buttermilk and set aside. In a heavy pan or wok, heat 4 tablespoons of the ghee over medium-high heat. When the ghee is hot but not smoking, use a slotted spatula to push small amounts of the remaining paste into the hot ghee. Small spongy balls will form. Cook in batches until the balls turn light brown on all sides; remove with a slotted spoon or spatula. Continue until no batter remains.

In another large, heavy pan, heat the remaining 2 tablespoons ghee over medium heat. Add the fenugreek seeds, chili peppers, and asafoetida. Mix in the remaining 4 cups buttermilk, and bring the mixture to a boil. At this point, the buttermilk will curdle or separate. Stirring constantly, add the reserved buttermilk and chick-pea paste mixture to bind the soup so it thickens nicely. Boil, uncovered, for 25 minutes over medium heat, stirring frequently. Reduce the heat and add the fried chick-pea balls. Cook, uncovered, for 45 minutes, stirring occasionally to prevent burning.

Just before serving combine the topping ingredients over low heat and pour 1 teaspoonful atop each bowl.

Serve with plain Basmati rice, a dry vegetable, and chapatis, puris, or parathas.

Variation
> Plain yogurt or soy yogurt, thinned with water, may be
> used instead of buttermilk.

Chick-pea Dumpling Soup

Serves 6

1 cup dried chick-peas, cleaned and soaked overnight
¹/₂ teaspoon salt
1 teaspoon Dal Masala (page 78)

Basic Soaked Masala:
¹/₂ cup water
1 teaspoon ground turmeric
2 teaspoons ground coriander.

2 tablespoons ghee, plus additional for shallow-frying
1 teaspoon fenugreek seeds
2 cloves garlic, sliced
4 medium onions, chopped
¹/₂ cup plain yogurt
4 medium potatoes, washed and cubed
¹/₂ teaspoon salt
3 cups water
1¹/₂ teaspoons Garam Masala (page 77)

Drain the chick-peas and discard the soaking water. Mash the chick-peas into a thick paste in a mortar. Whip with an egg beater until fluffy, or use a blender to combine these two steps. Add the salt and Dal Masala.

Soak the ingredients for the basic soaked masala for 5 minutes; stir into a thin paste and set aside.

Test the chick-pea paste by dropping a small amount of it into a cup of warm water. When the paste has been whipped enough, it floats and is ready to cook. Form the paste into cherry-size balls.

In a wok, heat enough ghee for shallow-frying. Drop five of the chick-pea balls into the hot ghee to form dumplings. Cook over medium heat until golden brown and remove. Repeat until all of the chick-pea balls are cooked.

In a heavy pan, heat the remaining 2 tablespoons of ghee. Add the fenugreek seeds and cook until browned. Add the garlic and onions and cook until the onions turn light brown. Add the soaked masala and cook until the ghee surfaces. Stir in the yogurt and cook until the ghee surfaces again. Add the dumplings, potatoes, salt, and water. Cook until the potatoes are soft, about 40 to 45 minutes. Remove from the heat and let stand for 5 minutes.

Stir in the Garam Masala and allow the flavors to blend for 10 minutes.

Serve with rice and/or any kind of Indian bread.

Moong Dal Dumpling Soup

Serves 4

1 cup whole moong or urad beans, cleaned, soaked overnight, and drained
1 teaspoon salt
1 teaspoon Garam Masala (page 77)
1 tablespoon ghee, plus additional for shallow-frying

Basic Soaked Masala:
¹/₂ cup water
1 teaspoon ground turmeric
2 teaspoons ground coriander

3 cloves garlic, thinly sliced
¹/₂ teaspoon fenugreek seeds
1 cup shelled fresh green peas
1 cup water
1 large potato, boiled and cubed (optional)
¹/₄ head of cauliflower, boiled and broken into florets (optional)
¹/₂ cup plain yogurt
4 medium onions, chopped and blended into a paste
1 teaspoon fennel seeds
8 whole black peppercorns
seeds of 1 black cardamom pod
1 teaspoon coriander seeds
5 bay leaves
1 teaspoon grated fresh ginger
1 cinnamon stick (2 to 3 inches long)

Mash the beans into a thick paste in a mortar. Whip the paste with an egg beater. (A blender can be used to combine these two steps.) Add the salt and Garam Masala to the paste.

Drop a small amount of the bean paste into a cup of water. If the paste floats, It is ready to cook; if not ready, whip the paste a bit more. Moisten your hands with a bit of oil and roll the paste into small, cherry-sized balls. Continue until no dough remains (it should make 20 to 24 balls).

In a heavy pan or wok, heat enough ghee for shallow-frying. Fry the dumplings in batches over medium heat until golden brown on all sides. Soak the cooked balls in hot water for 1 hour, then squeeze to remove all water. This step helps to remove excess fat and make the balls light and soft.

Combine the basic soaked masala ingredients and let stand for 5 minutes; stir the mixture into a thin paste and set aside.

In a deep soup pot, heat the remaining tablespoon of ghee and add garlic and fenugreek seeds and sauté until the garlic is lightly browned. Add the soaked masala and stir. Cook this mixture until the ghee surfaces. If the mixture becomes dry, add just enough water to keep it from sticking to the pot or burning. Add the dumplings, peas, and 1 cup water. (Potato and/or cauliflower pieces may be added at this point to supplement the dumplings, if desired.) Cook over low heat until half of the water has evaporated, about 25 to 30 minutes.

Mix in the yogurt, onions, and all of the remaining ingredients. Cover and cook over medium heat for 20 minutes. Season with about ¹/₂ teaspoon salt and let stand for 15 minutes to allow the flavors to blend.

Serve with parathas or rice.

Sprouted Black Chick-pea Soup

Serves 4

    1 cup whole black chick-peas (*kala chana*)
    2 to 3 cups water

Basic Soaked Masala with onion:
    1/2 cup water
    1 teaspoon ground turmeric
    2 teaspoons ground coriander
    1 small onion, grated

    2 tablespoons ghee
    4 medium onions, chopped
    3 cloves garlic, chopped
    1 large tomato, quartered
    3 medium potatoes, washed and cubed
    1 1/2 cups water
    1 teaspoon salt
    1 teaspoon ajwain seeds

Garam Masala (whole):
    2 whole black peppercorns (per person)
    4 whole cloves
    seeds of 1 black cardamom pod
    4 bay leaves, crushed
    2 cinnamon sticks (each 2 inches long)
    2 tablespoons grated fresh ginger

Clean and soak 1 cup of dried whole black chick-peas (*kala chana*) in a bowl with 2 to 3 cups water overnight. Place bowl in a warm, dark place for 1 to 2 days more, changing the water once or twice daily, and adding less water each time, until the sprouts are clearly visible on each bean.

To increase iron content of black chick-peas, they can be soaked in a cast-iron pot. This darkens the skins of the beans, adding to their already rich protein and mineral content.

Combine the basic soaked masala ingredients and let stand for 5 minutes; stir into a thin paste and set aside.

In a large wok, heat the ghee over medium heat. Sauté the onions and garlic until golden brown and the ghee surfaces. Add the soaked masala and simmer until the ghee surfaces again. Stir in the tomato and cook until dissolved. Add the sprouted chick-peas and the potato cubes, and simmer for 3 minutes. Add the water, salt, and ajwain seeds. Cover and cook over medium heat for 35 minutes, or until the sprouts and potatoes are soft but not quite tender.

Add the garam masala and cook for 10 minutes, or until all of the ingredients are tender.

Serve with chapatis or puris.

Black Chick-pea Soup with Masala

Serves 4

1 cup whole black chick-peas (*kala chana*), washed, soaked for 24 to
    36 hours, and drained
water to cover (for cooking)
1 teaspoon salt
1 teaspoon baking soda (optional, to soften beans)

Basic Soaked Masala:
    ½ cup water
    1 teaspoon ground turmeric
    2 teaspoons ground coriander

    2 cloves garlic, crushed
    1 large onion, grated

    4 tablespoons ghee
    2 large onions, sliced
    1 clove garlic, chopped
    1 tomato, quartered
    1 cup plain yogurt

In a heavy pan, bring the water to a boil. Add the beans, salt, and baking soda, cover, and cook over medium-high heat for 2 hours, or until the beans are soft.

Combine the basic soaked masala ingredients and let stand for 5 minutes; stir into a thin paste. Add the crushed garlic and grated onion to the soaked masala and set aside.

In a large cast-iron pot, heat the ghee over medium heat. Sauté the sliced onions and chopped garlic until golden brown and the ghee surfaces. Add the tomato and cook until dissolved. Stir in the soaked masala and continue cooking until the ghee resurfaces. Stir in the yogurt and simmer until the ghee surfaces a final time. Add the cooked black chick-peas.

Serve with any kind of salad and puris or chapatis.

Chick-pea Soup with Garam Masala

Serves 4

> 1 cup dried chick-peas (garbanzo beans/*kabli chana*), cleaned and
>   soaked for 24 to 36 hours
> water
> 1½ teaspoons salt
> 1 tablespoon ghee
> 1 teaspoon black cumin seeds
> 2 large onions, chopped
> 1 medium tomato, quartered

Garam Masala (whole):
> 8 whole black peppercorns
> 4 whole cloves
> seeds of 1 black cardamom pod
> 3 bay leaves, crumbled
> 1 to 2 tablespoons grated fresh ginger

Drain the chick-peas and reserve 1 cup of the soaking water.

In a heavy saucepan, combine the chick-peas with water to cover and bring to a boil. Add 1 teaspoon of the salt just before the water boils. Reduce the heat, cover, and cook over medium-high heat for 1½ hours, or until tender.

In another heavy saucepan, heat the ghee over medium heat. Add the cumin seeds and onions and cook until the ghee surfaces. Add the tomato and cook until dissolved. Stir in the cooked chick-peas, the reserved soaking water, and the remaining ½ teaspoon salt.

Stir in the garam masala. Cover and cook over medium heat for 10 minutes. Remove from the heat and allow the flavors to blend.

Serve with rice and Indian bread.

Split Moong Dal Soup

with Fenugreek Leaves

Serves 4

1 cup dried split and peeled moong beans, washed, soaked for 1 hour, and drained

a handful (about 4 tablespoons) of fenugreek (*methi*) leaves, soaked*

Tarka:

1 tablespoon ghee

¹/₂ teaspoon black cumin seeds

4 whole cloves

seeds of 1 black cardamom pod, ground

pinch of asafoetida powder

Prepare the moong beans according to the Basic Dal recipe (page 95). Add the fenugreek leaves after the first 15 minutes of cooking.

To prepare the tarka, heat the ghee in a ladle or small frying pan. Add the cumin seeds and sauté until well-toasted and fragrant. Add the sizzling tarka to the dal and cover immediately with a tight-fitting lid. Allow to stand for a few minutes, while the flavors are absorbed.

Serve with chapatis and a vegetable dish.

*Note: Dried fenugreek leaves should be soaked in water for 5 minutes and then stirred with the fingertips. The dust that settles to the bottom of the pan is not good to ingest and should be discarded. The clean, soaked leaves can be picked up with the fingers or removed with a slotted spoon.

Whole Moong Dal Soup
with Spices

Serves 4

4 cups water
½ teaspoon ground turmeric
¼ teaspoon ground coriander
½ teaspoon salt
1 cup dried whole moong beans, washed, soaked, and drained

Tarka:
1 tablespoon ghee
seeds of 1 black cardamom pod, crushed
1 dried red chili pepper, crushed
pinch of asafoetida powder

In a heavy pan, combine the water, turmeric, coriander, and salt and bring to a boil. Add the moong beans, cover, and cook over medium-high heat for 30 to 40 minutes, or until dal soften and can be easily mashed with a spoon.

To prepare the tarka, heat the ghee in a ladle or small frying pan. Add the spices and sauté for a few minutes, until well-toasted and fragrant. Add the sizzling tarka to the dal and cover immediately with a tight-fitting lid. Allow to stand for a few minutes, while the flavors blend.

Serve with rice and an Indian bread.

Whole Moong Dal Soup

with Dal Masala

Serves 4

    1 cup dried whole moong dal with skins
    4 cups cold water
    1 teaspoon ground turmeric
    2 teaspoons ground coriander
    1 teaspoon salt
    1 tomato, quartered and sliced
    1 teaspoon Dal Masala (page 78)

Tarka:
    1 tablespoon ghee
    2 to 4 cloves garlic, chopped

    Cumin Seed Dressing (page 94)

Prepare the dal according to the Basic Dal recipe on page 95. During the cooking process, add the tomato. When the dal is cooked, add the Dal Masala.

To prepare the tarka, heat the ghee in a ladle or small frying pan. Add the garlic and sauté for a few minutes, until well-toasted and fragrant. Add the sizzling tarka to the dal and cover immediately with a tight-fitting lid. Allow to stand for a few minutes, while flavors blend.

Top with the Cumin Seed Dressing and serve with rice and Indian bread.

Moongorhi with Mushrooms

Serves 2

Moongorhi are moong dal dumplings the size of hazelnuts. They are formed from a split moong bean and spice paste and sun-dried. These dried moongorhi balls can be kept for quite some time and used as needed. Delicious by themselves, they can also be prepared with potatoes, soy yogurt, or mushrooms. Moongorhi can be purchased ready-made in Indian groceries or ordered directly from India (see Sources of Supply, page 256).

Basic Soaked Masala:
2 tablespoons water
1/2 teaspoon ground turmeric
1 teaspoon ground coriander

1 tablespoon ghee
1 handful or 1/2 cup moongorhi balls
1 large onion, finely chopped
1 medium tomato, quartered
5 ounces chanterelle or other mushrooms, sliced
1 medium potato, peeled and cubed
3/4 teaspoon salt
2 cups hot water

Optional Masala (finely ground):
2 whole cloves
4 whole black peppercorns
seeds of 1 black cardamom pod, ground

Combine the basic soaked masala ingredients and let stand for 5 minutes; stir into a thin paste and set aside.

In a heavy pan, heat the ghee over low heat. Add moongorhi balls and sauté until golden brown on all sides. Remove from the pan and set aside. In the remaining ghee, sauté the onion until lightly browned and the ghee surfaces.

Add the soaked masala to the onion-ghee mixture and cook until the ghee surfaces again. Add the tomato and mushrooms, cover, and cook over medium heat until the tomato dissolves. Add the potato, moongorhi, salt, and hot water, and simmer for a few minutes more, until all of the ingredients become soft.

Add the optional masala, if desired.

Serve with chapatis or parathas and a dry, cooked vegetable dish.

Variation
The following vegetables can be added after the tomato: 2 tablespoons grated celery, 1 small grated beet, and /or 3 1/2 ounces fresh spinach leaves.

Urad Dal Soup with Tarka

Serves 4

Urad beans have a good taste, even when cooked without spices. To reduce problems with Wind, those who have weak stomachs can add fresh ginger to any urad dal dish.

> 4 cups water
> ¼ teaspoon ground turmeric
> ½ teaspoon ground coriander
> 1 teaspoon salt
> 1 cup split urad dal with skins, washed, soaked for 2 hours, and drained
> 1 piece (about 2 inches) fresh ginger, finely chopped

Tarka:
> 1 tablespoon ghee
> 2 to 3 cloves garlic, finely sliced
> seeds of 1 black cardamom pod
> 1 to 2 dried red chili peppers, crushed
> pinch of asafoetida powder

Onion Dressing:
> ¼ cup ghee
> 1 to 2 medium onions, chopped or thinly sliced

In a heavy pan, bring the water to a boil. Add the turmeric, coriander, salt, and soaked beans. Cover and cook over medium heat for 1 hour, or until soft. Reduce the heat and add the fresh ginger. Simmer for 5 minutes and remove from the heat.

To prepare the tarka, heat the ghee in a ladle or small frying pan. Add the garlic and tarka spices and sauté for a few minutes until well-toasted and fragrant. Add the sizzling tarka to the dal and cover immediately with a tight-fitting lid. Allow to stand for a few minutes, while the flavors blend.

To prepare the onion dressing, heat the ghee in a small frying pan. Sauté the onions until golden brown and divide among the servings of dal.

118

Urad Dal Soup
with Spinach and Fenugreek Leaves

Serves 4

4 cups water
1 teaspoon ground turmeric
2 teaspoons ground coriander
1 cup split and peeled urad dal, washed, soaked for 1 hour, and
   drained
8 ounces fresh spinach, washed well and stemmed
2 tablespoons dried fenugreek (*methi*) leaves, soaked*
1 piece (about 2 inches) fresh ginger, finely grated

Tarka:
1 tablespoon ghee
2 to 3 cloves garlic, finely sliced
seeds of 1 black cardamom pod
1 to 2 dried red chili peppers, crushed
pinch of asafoetida powder

Cumin Seed Dressing (page 94)

In a heavy pan, bring the water, turmeric, and coriander to a boil. Add the
soaked dal, spinach, and fenugreek, cover, and cook over medium heat for 1
hour, or until soft.

Reduce the heat and add the fresh ginger. Simmer for 5 minutes and remove from the heat.

To prepare the tarka, heat the ghee in a ladle or small frying pan. Add
the garlic and tarka spices and sauté for a few minutes, until well-toasted and
fragrant. Add the sizzling tarka to the dal and cover immediately with a tight-
fitting lid. Allow to stand for a few minutes, while the flavors blend.

Top each serving of dal with Cumin Seed Dressing and serve with rice.

*Note: Dried fenugreek leaves should be soaked in water for 5
       minutes and then stirred with the fingertips. The dust that
       settles to the bottom is not good to ingest and should be
       discarded.

Red Lentil Soup with Zucchini

Serves 4

2 cups water
1 teaspoon ground turmeric
2 teaspoons ground coriander
1 cup peeled and split red lentils (*masoor dal*), washed, soaked, and
    drained
2 small zucchini, cubed
1 teaspoon salt

Tarka:
1 tablespoon ghee
2 cloves garlic, sliced
1/8 teaspoon black cumin seeds
1 small dried red chili pepper, crushed
1/4 teaspoon asafoetida powder

In a heavy pan, bring the water, turmeric, and coriander to a boil. Stir in the lentils, zucchini, and salt. Cover and cook over medium heat for 1 hour, or until soft.

To prepare the tarka, heat the ghee in a ladle or small frying pan. Add the garlic and tarka spices and sauté until garlic and cumin seeds are well-toasted and fragrant. Add the sizzling tarka to the dal and cover immediately with a tight-fitting lid. Allow to stand for a few minutes, while the flavors blend.

Serve with rice and an Indian bread and ginger pickle.

Red Lentil Soup with Leek and Beet

Serves 4

    4 cups water
    1 teaspoon ground turmeric
    2 teaspoons ground coriander
    2 medium leeks, cleaned and the whites chopped
    1 medium beet, cleaned, peeled, and grated
    1 cup red lentils (*masoor dal*), washed, soaked, and drained
    1 teaspoon salt
    1 cup soy yogurt
    1 medium tomato, quartered
    Onion Dressing (page 93)

In a heavy pan, bring the water, turmeric, and coriander to a boil. Add the leeks and beet and boil for 10 minutes.

Stir in the lentils and salt and bring to a boil again. Add the soy yogurt and tomato, and cook for 10 minutes more.

Cover and cook over medium-low heat for 40 minutes.

Top with Onion Dressing and serve with rice, vegetable, and an Indian bread.

Urad Dal Dumplings in Yogurt

Serves 5

½ cup split and peeled urad dal, washed, soaked overnight, and drained

Masala:
   ½ teaspoon ground ginger
   ½ teaspoon ground cumin
   ¼ teaspoon salt

½ cup ghee
1 cup plain yogurt
1 cup water
1 teaspoon salt
1 teaspoon Garam Masala (page 77), or Tarka (see Bean Balls in Yogurt recipe, page 102)

Mash the urad dal to a fine paste in a mortar or blender. Add the masala mixture and mix well. Form small balls the size of cherries with teaspoonfuls of this paste.

In a wok, heat the ghee until it is hot but not smoking. Deep-fry the balls in batches over low heat, turning to cook evenly, until golden brown. Remove the dumplings from the wok and place in a bowl of hot water for 30 minutes.

In a separate bowl, combine the yogurt and 1 cup water and beat with a fork until foamy. Add the salt and either the Garam Masala or Tarka.

Drain the dumplings, squeezing carefully to remove excess water. Gently drop into the yogurt mixture.

Serve with saunth.

Arwi Root (Taro) Soup with Lentils

4 cups water
4 medium arwi roots (taro), cleaned, peeled, and cut in ¹/₂-inch slices
1 teaspoon ground turmeric
2 teaspoons ground coriander
1 cup red lentils, cleaned and soaked overnight
1 teaspoon salt
1 teaspoon Dal Masala (page 78)

Tarka:
1 tablespoon ghee
4 to 6 cloves garlic, finely chopped
¹/₂ teaspoon black cumin seeds
1 teaspoon sesame seeds
¹/₄ teaspoon asafoetida powder

Apply mustard oil to the hands to avoid a tingling sensation in the fingertips from peeling the arwi root.

Drain the lentils and discard the soaking water. In a saucepan, bring the 4 cups water to a boil. Add the arwi root, turmeric, and coriander. Reduce the heat, cover, and cook for 30 minutes, or until the arwi is soft.

Add the lentils and salt and continue to cook over medium heat for 45 minutes, or until the lentils are soft and about half the water remains.

Remove from the heat and add the Dal Masala.

To make the tarka, heat the ghee in a ladle or small frying pan. Add the garlic and tarka spices and sauté until well-toasted and fragrant. Add the sizzling tarka to the soup and cover immediately with a tight-fitting lid. Allow to stand for a few minutes while the flavors blend.

Serve with rice and any kind of Indian bread—puris, chapatis, or parathas.

Potato Soup with Cumin Seeds

Serves 4

12 very small (walnut-sized) potatoes, washed
2 tablespoons ghee
1 teaspoon black cumin seeds
1 dried red chili pepper, crushed (optional)
1 teaspoon salt
1 small tomato, quartered
4 to 5 cups hot water
1 teaspoon fresh coriander leaves (optional)

Boil the potatoes until cooked but still firm; drain, peel, and set aside.

In a heavy pot, heat the ghee over medium heat. Add the cumin seeds and chili pepper and roast until the cumin seeds pop. Add the potatoes, salt, and tomato and stir carefully for a few minutes. Add the hot water, cover, and cook for 5 minutes.

Remove from the heat, and garnish with the coriander.

Serve with chapatis or parathas and a vegetable dish.

Yellow Lentil Soup with Sour Taste

Serves 4

4 cups water
1 cup yellow lentils (*toor dal*), washed, soaked for 2 hours, and
    drained
1 teaspoon ground turmeric
2 teaspoons ground coriander
1 large tomato, quartered
1 cup fresh whey (if available), or 1 teaspoon dried mango powder
1 teaspoon salt
Onion Dressing (page 93)

In a heavy pan, bring the water, turmeric, and coriander to a boil. Add the lentils and bring back to a boil. Stir in the tomato, whey or mango powder, and salt and boil for 10 to 15 minutes (longer if whey is added). Reduce the heat to medium-low, cover, and cook for 45 minutes.

Top with the Onion Dressing and serve with rice, a vegetable, and an Indian bread.

Whole Moong Dal Soup
with Yogurt

Serves 4

4 cups water
½ teaspoon ground turmeric
1 teaspoon ground coriander
1 teaspoon salt
½ cup plain yogurt
2 tablespoons jaggery (optional)
1 cup dried whole moong beans, washed, soaked, and drained

Garam Masala (whole):
8 whole peppercorns
4 whole cloves
seeds of 1 black cardamom pod
pinch of ground cinnamon

Tarka:
1 tablespoon ghee
pinch asafoetida powder

In a cast-iron pot, bring the water to a boil. Add the turmeric, coriander, salt, yogurt, and jaggery (if desired), and continue boiling for 20 to 25 minutes. Add the moong beans and boil another 5 to 10 minutes. Cover and cook over medium heat for 45 minutes, or until the dal softens.

Meanwhile, preheat the oven to 400 degrees F.

Add the garam masala and stir well. Tightly cover the pot and bake for 25 minutes. Remove from the oven and allow to cool, covered, for 15 minutes.

To prepare the tarka, heat the ghee in a ladle or small frying pan. Add the asafoetida and sauté for a few minutes, until fragrant. Add the sizzling tarka to the dal and cover immediately with a tight-fitting lid. Allow to stand for a few minutes, while the flavors blend.

Serve with rice and an Indian bread.

Potato Soup

with Onions and Red Pepper

Serves 2

1 tablespoon ghee
1 large onion, chopped
1 dried red chili pepper, crushed
2 large potatoes, scrubbed and cubed
³/₄ teaspoon salt
2 cups hot water
fresh coriander leaves (optional)

In a heavy pan, warm the ghee over medium heat. Add the onion and sauté until golden brown and the ghee surfaces. Add the chili pepper and roast until the color darkens. Mix in the potatoes and salt. Add the hot water, cover, and simmer for 25 to 30 minutes, or until potatoes are soft.

Garnish with the fresh coriander leaves, if desired. Serve with chapatis or parathas and a second vegetable dish.

Chapter Four

SAVORY RICE DISHES

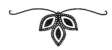

Rice with Cumin

Serves 2 to 4

2 to 3 tablespoons ghee
1 teaspoon black cumin seeds, cleaned
1 dried red chili pepper, crushed
2 medium onions, chopped
2 to 3 medium carrots, finely grated (optional)
1 cup Basmati rice, cleaned and rinsed
2 cups water
1 teaspoon salt

In a large, deep frying pan or saucepan, heat the ghee over medium heat. Add the cumin seeds and chili pepper and sauté until the cumin seeds pop and release their aroma. Add the onions and sauté until golden brown. Add the carrots and cook, stirring constantly, for 10 minutes. Mix in the rice and cook, stirring, for 3 minutes. Add the water and bring to a boil. Reduce the heat and add the salt. Cover and simmer until every grain of rice is well done, about 30 minutes.

Meanwhile, preheat the oven to 450 degrees F.

Place the tightly covered pan in the oven and turn off the heat. Allow to sit for 5 to 10 minutes to absorb excess moisture.

Serve with raita, pickles, and pappadams.

Variation

Other vegetables such as cauliflower, peas, grated beets, or finely chopped cabbage can be substituted for the carrots.

Coconut Rice

Serves 2 to 4

1 cup Basmati rice, cleaned and rinsed
2 to 4 tablespoons grated coconut, fresh or dried
2 whole cloves
2 cups water

Soak the rice for 1 hour; drain.

In a saucepan, combine the rice, coconut, cloves, and water and bring to a boil. Reduce the heat, cover, and simmer for 20 minutes.

Meanwhile, preheat the oven to 450 degrees F.

Place the tightly covered pan of rice in the oven and turn off the heat. Allow to sit for 5 to 10 minutes to absorb excess moisture.

Serve hot, with dal and a vegetable of your choice.

Rice with Basic Masala (Tahiri)

Serves 4

1 cup rice, cleaned and rinsed
2 to 3 tablespoons ghee
1 teaspoon fenugreek seeds
1 teaspoon black cumin seeds
2 cloves garlic, chopped
2 medium onions, chopped
1 teaspoon ground turmeric
1 teaspoon ground coriander
1 medium tomato, chopped
1¼ shelled fresh peas
½ cup cauliflower florets
2 large potatoes, peeled and cubed
2 cups water
1 teaspoon salt

Masala:
8 whole black peppercorns
4 whole cloves
seeds of 1 black cardamom pod

Soak the rice in water to cover for 30 minutes; rinse and pat dry.

In a saucepan, heat the ghee over medium heat. Add the fenugreek seeds, cumin seeds, and garlic, and sauté until the garlic is browned. Add the onions and cook until golden brown. Add the turmeric, coriander, and tomato, and cook over medium heat until the ghee surfaces. Add the rice and stir for 2 minutes. Add the peas, cauliflower, and potatoes, and cook for 2 minutes. Stir in water and salt and bring to a boil. Immediately reduce the heat and stir in the masala. Cover and simmer for 30 to 40 minutes, or until the water is absorbed by the rice.

Meanwhile, preheat the oven to 450 degrees F.

Place the tightly covered pan in the oven and turn off the heat. Allow to sit for 5 to 10 minutes to absorb excess moisture.

Serve with a raita, chutney, pickles, and pappadams.

Lentil Kababs Pulao

Serves 6

1 cup red lentils (*masoor dal*), cleaned, soaked overnight, and rinsed
5 tablespoons ghee
1 teaspoon Garam Masala (page 77)

Basic Soaked Masala:
$^1/_2$ cup water
1 teaspoon ground turmeric
2 teaspoons ground coriander

6 medium onions, chopped
2 medium tomatoes, quartered
1 cup Basmati rice, cleaned and soaked in water to cover for 1 hour
2 cups water
$^1/_2$ cup fresh or frozen peas
1 teaspoon salt
12 whole black peppercorns
6 whole cloves
seeds of $1^1/_2$ black cardamom pods
$^1/_4$ teaspoon ground cinnamon
6 bay leaves

To prepare lentil balls, grind the lentils in a mortar. Whip the mixture into a paste with an egg beater. (A blender can be used to combine these two steps.)

Heat 1 tablespoon of the ghee in a skillet or wok over medium-low heat. When the ghee is hot but not smoking, drop in the entire paste mixture. Stir with a spatula and cook over low heat until the mixture thickens and changes color. Turn off the heat and stir in the Garam Masala. Allow the paste to cool, and form it into 1-inch balls.

Combine the basic soaked masala ingredients and let stand for 5 minutes; stir to form a thin paste and set aside.

In a heavy pan or wok, heat the remaining 4 tablespoons ghee. Add the onions and sauté until light brown. Add the soaked masala and cook until the ghee surfaces. Add the tomatoes, cover, and cook until they are completely dissolved. Add the lentil balls, and simmer for 5 minutes. Add the rice, and stir for 5 minutes. Add the water and bring to a boil. Mix in the peas. Finely grind all of the remaining spices and add them to the mixture. Cover and cook over low heat until all the water is absorbed, about 30 to 35 minutes.

Meanwhile, preheat the oven to 450 degrees F.

Place the tightly covered pan in the oven and turn off the heat. Allow to sit 5 to 10 minutes to absorb excess moisture.

Serve with pickles and pappadams.

KHICHARIS

In general, khichari is good for children, the infirmed, and older people. The combination of rice with dal makes a complete balanced protein. Typically served as a midday meal in an Indian home, this dish does not take long to cook and is delicious and satisfying. While khichari is most often prepared with moong beans, urad beans , or *chana dal* (split chick-peas), other dal are also used—soybeans, split peas, or lentils. If possible, dal with skins should be used because of the increased vitamin content and roughage the skins provide.

In the preparation of khichari, the dal is soaked for no more than an hour. Though the dal takes a little longer to cook, it retains a firmer texture, which is desirable in khichari.

Moong dal khichari is ideal for people who suffer from chronic dysentery or peptic ulcers. It is also good for those who cannot digest properly, for those doing spiritual practices who need to eat simple but nourishing foods, or for those who must avoid fried foods. By increasing the proportion of dal in the khichari, as in the following recipe, the dish becomes more fortifying and subdues Kapha.

Moong Dal Khichari

Serves 2 to 3

> 1 cup Basmati rice
> 1¹/₂ cups split moong beans with skins
> 8 cups water, for cooking
> ³/₄ teaspoon salt
> 1 beet, grated (optional)
> 2 tablespoons ghee
> ¹/₂ teaspoon black cumin seeds

Combine the rice and dal in a large bowl and add enough water to cover. Soak for 1 hour. Drain, wash, and rinse the mixture. Place it in a heavy pan and add the 8 cups of water and the salt. Cover tightly and bring to a boil over medium heat. Stir in grated beet, if desired. Reduce the heat and simmer for 30 minutes.

Meanwhile, preheat the oven to 450 degrees F.

Place the tightly covered pan of cooked khichari in the oven and turn off the heat. Allow to sit for 5 to 10 minutes to absorb excess moisture.

In a small frying pan, warm the ghee over medium heat. Add the cumin seeds and sauté until brown and fragrant. Serve the khichari hot, topped with this dressing.

For those with stomach problems, this dish can be accompanied by lemon pickle* and yogurt or buttermilk. Healthy people can eat this dish with pappadam (dal wafers) and chutneys or pickles.

*Note: In general, rice and lemon juice is not a good combination. Lemon pickle with dal, however, is quite a different matter; it works like a medicine for the stomach.

Red Lentil Khichari with Beets

Serves 1 to 2

1/3 cup **Basmati rice**
1/3 cup **split and peeled red lentils**
2 cups **water**
1/2 teaspoon **salt**
1 medium **beet, peeled and grated**

Masala (advisable in winter):
1 tablespoon **grated fresh ginger**
2 whole **cloves**
4 whole **black peppercorns**
seeds of 1 **black cardamom pod**

Combine the rice and red lentils in a pan and soak in water to cover for one hour.

Drain, wash, and rinse the rice and lentils. Combine the mixture with the 2 cups of water and the salt. Cover and bring to a boil over medium heat. With a tablespoon, skim off and discard the white foam that surfaces. Add the grated beet and masala mixture, if desired. Stir and let return to a boil. Cover and simmer over low heat for 30 minutes.

Meanwhile, preheat the oven to 450 degrees F.

Place the tightly covered pan of cooked khichari in the oven and turn off the heat. Allow to sit for 5 to 10 minutes to absorb excess moisture. If time does not permit, simply cook, uncovered, for a few more minutes.

This dish can be topped with a teaspoon (or tablespoon) of hot ghee per person and either 1/8 teaspoon cumin seeds, roasted, or 1/2 small, chopped onion, sautéed until golden brown and crisp, per person.

Serve hot with pappadam. In summer, yogurt, buttermilk, or a raita make an ideal combination with khichari.

Dalia Khichari

Serves 2 to 4

Ideal for health-oriented people or bodybuilders, this dish can also be eaten by sick people, if the nuts and poppy seeds are omitted. It is beneficial for mucus-dominated individuals (Kaphas). Dalia Khichari can be taken by those suffering from a cold, in which case white poppy seeds should be used.

½ cup split moong beans with skins, cleaned and rinsed
½ cup cracked wheat (*∂alia*)
1 tablespoon ghee
1½ teaspoons white cumin seeds, cleaned
1 whole dried red chili pepper (optional)
¼ teaspoon asafoetida powder
3 cups water
¾ teaspoon salt
½ cup cashews, almonds (soaked overnight and peeled),
   or pine nuts, soaked in water overnight and finely ground

Masala:
6 whole black peppercorns
3 whole cloves
seeds of 1 black cardamom pod
2 tablespoons white or black poppy seeds soaked overnight and finely
   ground (optional)

Mix the moong beans with the cracked wheat and soak in water to cover for 1 hour. Drain and discard the soaking water.

In a large, heavy pan, heat the ghee over medium heat. Add the cumin seeds, chili pepper, and asafoetida and sauté until toasted. Mix in the beans and cracked wheat along with the 3 cups of water and bring to a boil. Add the salt, nuts, and masala. Cover and simmer over low heat for 30 to 45 minutes, or until the beans are soft.

Serve with pappadam, chutney, and any pickle.

Pulao with Peas

Serves 4

1 cup Basmati rice, cleaned and rinsed
water to cover
2 to 3 tablespoons ghee
1 teaspoon black cumin seeds
1 medium clove garlic, chopped
2 medium onions, chopped
1 pound (³/₄ to 1 cup) fresh peas in the pod, shelled
2 cups hot water
1 teaspoon salt
4 whole cloves
8 whole black peppercorns
seeds of 1 black cardamom pod
seeds of 2 green cardamom pods
1 stick (about 2 inches) cinnamon
4 bay leaves
pinch of ground nutmeg
1 piece (about 2 inches) fresh ginger, grated

Soak the rice in water to cover for 45 minutes. Drain and pat dry.

In a large heavy pan, heat ghee over medium heat. Add the cumin and garlic and sauté until browned. Add the onions and cook until golden brown. Add the rice and stir over low heat for 2 minutes. Stir in the peas and cook for 2 minutes. Add the hot water, salt, and all of the spices and mix well. Add the ginger and bring the mixture to a boil. Reduce the heat immediately, cover, and simmer until the water is absorbed, about 20 to 25 minutes.

Meanwhile, preheat the oven to 450 degrees F.

Place the tightly covered pan in the oven and turn off the heat. Allow to sit for 5 to 10 minutes to absorb excess moisture.

Serve with a raita, pappadams, chutney, and pickles.

Variation 1

Substitute paneer for half of the peas.

Variation 2

Add ¹/₂ cup of presoaked almonds, cashews, pine nuts, and walnuts, along with ¹/₄ cup raisins and ¹/₄ cup grated coconut. The nuts should be soaked together overnight and the almonds peeled after soaking. In winter, a pinch of saffron can be added to any pulao.

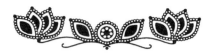

Chapter Five

VEGETABLE DISHES

Boiled Arwi Root (Taro)

Serves 4

> 6 medium arwi roots (taro), cleaned
> 3 tablespoons mustard oil, other vegetable oil, or ghee
> 6 cloves garlic, sliced
> 1 to 2 dried red chili peppers
> 6 large onions, chopped
> 1 teaspoon ajwain seeds
> 1 teaspoon salt

In a saucepan, cover the arwi roots with water and boil until soft. Peel the arwi and cut into small pieces.

In a frying pan, heat the oil over medium heat. Sauté the garlic and chili peppers until browned. Add the onions and sauté until golden. Add the arwi root, ajwain seeds, and salt. Cover and simmer over medium heat for 10 minutes.

Serve with rice and chapatis or puris.

Sautéed Arwi Root (Taro)

Serves 4

mustard oil (to lightly coat hands)
6 arwi roots (taro), cleaned and peeled

Basic Soaked Masala:
   ½ cup water
   1 teaspoon ground turmeric
   2 teaspoons ground coriander

   3 tablespoons ghee
   1 teaspoon fenugreek seeds
   3 cloves garlic, chopped
   6 medium onions, chopped (or weight equivalent to arwi)
   1 teaspoon ajwain seeds

Garam Masala (whole):
   8 whole black peppercorns
   4 whole cloves
   seeds of 2 black cardamom pods

   4 bay leaves
   pinch of ground cinnamon
   1 teaspoon salt

Apply mustard oil to hands to avoid a tingling sensation in the fingertips from peeling the arwi root. Peel and cut roots into ½-inch pieces.

Combine the basic soaked masala ingredients and let stand for 5 minutes; stir into a thin paste.

In a medium saucepan, heat the ghee and sauté the fenugreek and garlic over medium heat until the garlic turns brown. Add the onions and cook until golden brown. Add the ajwain seeds and soaked masala, and cook for 4 to 5 minutes, or until the ghee surfaces. Add the arwi root, cover, and cook until soft, about 40 to 45 minutes.

Stir in the garam masala, bay leaves, cinnamon, and salt, and remove from the heat. Allow the dish to stand, covered, for 5 minutes before serving.

Serve with rice and any kind of Indian bread—puris, chapatis, or parathas.

Dry Arwi Root (Taro) with Yogurt

Serves 4

> **6 medium (or 4 large) arwi roots (taro)**
> **2 to 3 tablespoons ghee**
> **1 teaspoon fenugreek seeds**
> **1 teaspoon black cumin seeds**
> **1 cup plain yogurt**
> **2 to 3 medium onions (or half the weight of the arwi roots), chopped**
> **1 teaspoon salt**

Cover the arwi roots with water and boil until soft, about 40 to 45 minutes. Allow to cool; peel and cut into 1-inch cubes.

In a heavy pan, heat the ghee over medium-high heat. Add the fenugreek seeds, cumin seeds, and yogurt, and cook, stirring occasionally so that the yogurt does not burn, for 20 minutes.

Add the arwi, onions, and salt and cook, stirring occasionally, for 20 minutes.

Serve with any kind of Indian bread—puris, chapatis, or parathas.

Red Beets with Peas

Serves 4

Basic Soaked Masala:
> **¹/₂ cup water**
> **1 teaspoon ground turmeric**
> **2 teaspoons ground coriander**

> **3 tablespoons ghee**
> **3 medium onions, chopped**
> **1 medium tomato, quartered**
> **2 medium red beets, scrubbed and thinly sliced**
> **1 teaspoon salt**
> **4 bay leaves**
> **6¹/₂ ounces (1 cup) shelled fresh or frozen green peas**
> **¹/₂ teaspoon ground cinnamon**

Garam Masala (finely ground):
> **8 whole black peppercorns**
> **4 whole cloves**
> **seeds of 1 black cardamom pod**

Combine the basic soaked masala ingredients and let stand for 5 minutes; stir into a thin paste and set aside.

In a heavy pan, heat the ghee over medium heat. Sauté the onions until light brown. Add the soaked masala and cook until the ghee surfaces. Mix in the tomato and cook until dissolved. Add the beets, salt, bay leaves, and peas, and simmer until the beets are soft, about 35 to 40 minutes.

Remove from the heat and stir in the cinnamon and garam masala.

Serve with puris or parathas.

Red Beets with Tomatoes

Serves 2

2 large red beets, well scrubbed

Basic Soaked Masala:
  ¹/₂ cup water
  1 teaspoon ground turmeric
  2 teaspoons ground coriander

  2 tablespoons mustard or other vegetable oil, or ghee
  1 clove garlic, chopped
  1 large onion, chopped
  2 small tomatoes, cubed
  ¹/₂ teaspoon salt

Garam Masala (finely ground):
  5 whole black peppercorns
  1 cinnamon stick (1 inch long)
  seeds of 1 black cardamom pod
  2 whole cloves

In a saucepan, cover the beets with water and boil until soft, about 40 to 45 minutes. Drain; when cooled, peel and thinly slice.

Combine the basic soaked masala ingredients and let stand for 5 minutes; stir into a thin paste and set aside.

In a heavy pan, heat the oil over medium heat. Add the garlic and onion and sauté until the oil surfaces. Add the soaked masala and cook until the oil surfaces again. Add the tomatoes and cook until dissolved, about 10 to 15 minutes. Add the beets, salt, and garam masala. Stir once and simmer over low heat for a few minutes. Turn off the heat and allow the flavors to blend.

Serve with dal and Indian bread (chapatis or parathas).

Cabbage "Purée"

Serves 4

  2 tablespoons mustard oil or other vegetable oil
  4 cloves garlic, finely chopped
  1 teaspoon fenugreek seeds
  1 whole dried red chili pepper
  1 medium green cabbage, cored and finely shredded
  1 teaspoon salt

In a wok, heat the oil over medium heat. Add the garlic and sauté until lightly browned. Add the fenugreek seeds and chili pepper and cook until well roasted. Stir in the cabbage and salt, cover, and simmer until the cabbage is soft and the oil surfaces.

Serve with a dal, raita, and chapatis.

Dry Bitter Melon (Karela)

Serves 2

Basic Soaked Masala:
> $^1/_2$ **cup water**
> $^1/_2$ **teaspoon ground turmeric**
> **1 teaspoon ground coriander**
> $^1/_2$ **teaspoon ground cumin**

> **1 tablespoon seedless tamarind pulp**
> $^1/_2$ **cup hot water**
> $2^1/_2$ **teaspoons jaggery**
> $^1/_2$ **cup water**
> **1 tablespoon ghee**
> **2 large onions (or double the amount of soaked *karela*), chopped**
> **1 handful ($^1/_2$ cup) dried bitter melon (*karela*), soaked in water to cover for 1 to 2 hours and drained**
> $^1/_2$ **teaspoon salt**
> $^3/_4$ **teaspoon anise seeds**
> $^3/_4$ **teaspoon fennel seeds**

> $^1/_2$ **teaspoon Garam Masala (page 77) (optional)**

Combine the soaked masala ingredients and let stand for 5 minutes; stir the mixture into a thin paste and set aside.

Soak the tamarind pulp in the hot water. Soak the jaggery in the water.

In a wok, heat the ghee over medium heat. Add the onions and sauté until brown and the ghee surfaces. Stir in the soaked masala and cook until ghee surfaces again. Add the karela, salt, and anise and fennel seeds, and mix well. Cover and simmer over low heat for 10 to 15 minutes.

Pour the tamarind and jaggery mixtures through a sieve into the pan and stir gently. Cook over medium heat until the karela is soft and the excess liquid evaporates, about 40 to 45 minutes.

Remove from the heat and add the Garam Masala.

Serve with chapatis and a leafy or soupy vegetable.

Sweet and Sour Bitter Melon (Karela)

Serves 4

pinch of salt
2 to 4 medium bitter melons (*karela*), cleaned and thinly sliced

Basic Soaked Masala:
 ¹/₂ cup water
 1 teaspoon ground turmeric
 2 teaspoons ground coriander
 1 teaspoon ground cumin

 1 teaspoon seedless tamarind pulp
 ¹/₄ cup hot water
 2 to 3 tablespoons jaggery
 2 tablespoons water
 3 tablespoons ghee
 2 large onions (or twice the weight of the bitter melon)
 1 teaspoon anise seeds
 1 teaspoon fennel seeds
 1 teaspoon salt
 1 teaspoon Garam Masala (page 77)

Add the pinch of salt to the fresh, thinly sliced bitter melon and set aside in a warm place for 1 to 2 days (in the summer, 24 hours will suffice). Discard the bitter water that drains from the melon.

Combine the basic soaked masala ingredients and let stand for 5 minutes; stir to form a thin paste and set aside.

Soak the tamarind pulp in the hot water for 15 minutes, or until soft. Press through a sieve to remove any solids.

Soak the jaggery in the 2 tablespoons water for 15 minutes.

In a heavy pan or wok, heat the ghee over medium heat. Add the onions and sauté until golden brown. Add the basic soaked masala and simmer until the ghee surfaces. Add the bitter melon and cook until the ghee surfaces again. Stir in the anise and fennel seeds, salt, tamarind liquid, and jaggery liquid. Cook until the bitter melon is soft and the ghee surfaces again, about 30 to 35 minutes. Remove from the heat, stir in the Garam Masala, and set aside for 5 to 10 minutes to allow the flavors to be absorbed.

Serve with parathas.

Broccoli and Mushroom Curry

Serves 6

Basic Soaked Masala:
 ¹/₂ cup water
 1 teaspoon ground turmeric
 2 teaspoons ground coriander
 1 teaspoon ground cumin

2 tablespoons ghee
3 large onions, chopped
1 whole large red chili pepper
1 pound fresh mushrooms, washed and sliced, or 12 ounces dried
   mushrooms, soaked in water for 2 hours
1 pound broccoli, cut into florets
1 teaspoon salt
12 whole black peppercorns
1 whole clove
pinch of ground cinnamon
seeds of 1½ black cardamom pods

Combine the ingredients for the basic soaked masala and let stand for 5 minutes; stir into a thin paste and set aside.

In a heavy pan, heat the ghee over medium heat. Add the onions and sauté until soft. Mix in the chili pepper and basic soaked masala, and cook until the ghee surfaces. Add the mushrooms, and simmer until the ghee resurfaces. Add the broccoli, salt, and all of the remaining spices. Cover and cook over low heat, stirring several times, until the ghee surfaces once more.

Stir and let flavors blend.

Serve with parathas.

Broccoli Stems
with Potatoes and Rice Cream

Serves 4

4 to 5 broccoli stalks, peeled and cut into 1½-inch pieces
¼ cup water
1 teaspoon ground turmeric
2 teaspoons ground coriander
1 teaspoon salt
3 large potatoes, peeled and quartered

3 tablespoons ghee
4 cloves garlic, sliced
1 teaspoon fenugreek seeds
1 onion, thinly sliced
2 to 3 tablespoons rice flour

In a heavy pan, combine the broccoli and water and bring to a boil. Reduce the heat and add the turmeric, coriander, salt, and potatoes. Cook until vegetables are soft and water is almost all evaporated, about 20 to 25 minutes.

In a heavy pan, heat ghee over medium heat. Add the garlic, fenugreek seeds, and onion, and sauté until the onion browns, about 10 to 15 minutes. Add the vegetable mixture.

Make a rice paste by mixing the rice flour with 1 tablespoon of water, so the consistency is slightly thicker than honey. Add the rice paste to the vegetable mixture and cook for 15 minutes. The addition of rice paste will make the broccoli crisp and tasty.

Serve with puris or parathas.

Cabbage with Carrots and Potatoes

Serves 4

2 tablespoons mustard oil or other vegetable oil
4 cloves garlic, finely chopped
1 teaspoon fenugreek seeds
1 whole dried red chili pepper
1 medium green cabbage, cored and finely shredded
4 to 5 medium carrots, thinly sliced
2 large potatoes, peeled and cubed
2 tablespoons dried fenugreek (*methi*) leaves, soaked in water for 5 to
   10 minutes*
1 teaspoon salt
1 teaspoon whole coriander seed
1 piece (about 1 inch long) fresh ginger, grated

In a heavy wok, heat the oil over medium heat. Add the garlic and sauté until light brown. Add the fenugreek seeds and chili pepper and roast for 2 to 3 minutes.

   Add the cabbage, carrots, and potatoes. Remove the fenugreek leaves from the soaking water by hand, and add to the vegetables. Stir in the salt, coriander seed, and ginger and cook, stirring frequently, until the vegetables are soft and the oil surfaces.

   Serve with chapatis or puris and tomato raita.

*Note: Dried fenugreek leaves should be soaked in water for 5 minutes and then stirred with the fingertips. The dust that settles to the bottom is not good to ingest and should be discarded.

Red Cabbage with Mushrooms

Serves 4

Basic Soaked Masala:
   ½ cup water
   1 teaspoon ground turmeric
   2 teaspoons ground coriander
   1 teaspoon ground cumin

3 tablespoons ghee
3 cloves garlic, sliced
1 teaspoon fenugreek seeds
4 large onions, sliced
1 medium tomato, quartered
1 medium red cabbage, cored and finely shredded
10 ounces fresh mushrooms, sliced, or 8 ounces dried mushrooms,
   soaked in water for 1 to 1½ hours

1 teaspoon salt
1 piece (¹/₂ to 1 inch long) fresh ginger, grated
¹/₂ teaspoon ground cinnamon
1 teaspoon Garam Masala (page 77)

Combine the ingredients for the basic soaked masala and let stand for 5 minutes; stir mixture into a thin paste and set aside.

In a heavy wok, heat the ghee over medium heat. Add the garlic and fenugreek seeds and sauté until light brown. Add the onions and cook until the ghee surfaces.

Add the soaked masala and tomato to the onion mixture, and sauté until the tomatoes dissolve and the ghee surfaces again. Add the cabbage, stir, and cook for 10 to 15 minutes.

Mix in the mushrooms and salt and stir well. Cover and simmer until the vegetables are soft, about 40 to 45 minutes. If too much liquid remains, remove the lid to allow the water to evaporate.

Remove from the heat and stir in the ginger, cinnamon, and Garam Masala. Allow flavors to blend and serve.

Cabbage with Onions

Serves 4

2 tablespoons mustard oil or other vegetable oil
4 cloves garlic, finely chopped
1 teaspoon fenugreek seeds
1 medium green cabbage, cored and shredded
1 teaspoon salt
4 large onions, chopped
1 teaspoon ground coriander
1 teaspoon ground cumin

Masala (whole):
1 tablespoon grated fresh ginger
¹/₄ teaspoon ground cinnamon
pinch of ground nutmeg
8 whole black peppercorns
4 whole cloves
seeds of 1 black cardamom pod

In a heavy wok, heat the oil over medium heat. Add the garlic and sauté until browned. Add the fenugreek seeds and roast for a few minutes. Mix in the cabbage and salt. Stir well and layer the onions over the cabbage. Cover and simmer over medium heat until the cabbage is tender and the oil surfaces, about 40 minutes.

Add the coriander and cumin and turn off the heat. Blend in the prepared masala and allow the flavors to blend.

This dish can be served with puris and kadhi or with a dal and chapatis or parathas.

Cabbage Rolls

Serves 4

1 medium green cabbage

Basic Soaked Masala:
   1/2 cup water
   1 teaspoon ground turmeric
   2 teaspoons ground coriander

2 tablespoons ghee
1 teaspoon fenugreek seeds
5 to 6 large onions, chopped
2 medium tomatoes, quartered
1 teaspoon fennel seeds
1 teaspoon salt
1 teaspoon Garam Masala (page 77)

Remove the leaves from the cabbage one by one, keeping them whole. Wash but do not cut the leaves. Remove the hard vein from each leaf.

Combine the ingredients for the basic soaked masala and let stand for 5 minutes; stir mixture into a thin paste and set aside.

In a heavy wok, heat the ghee over medium heat. Add the fenugreek seeds and sauté until brown. Add the onions and sauté until light brown and the ghee surfaces. Add the soaked masala to the wok and sauté until the ghee surfaces again. Mix in the tomatoes, cover, and simmer until dissolved.

Overlap two parts of cabbage leaf, and place 1 tablespoon of the filling on it. Roll as you would roll a cigarette, and tie a thread around it. Continue until all of the filling is used.

Carefully transfer the prepared cabbage rolls to another wok or pan, adding enough water to cover the rolls. Add the fennel seeds and salt. Simmer, uncovered, over low heat until the cabbage rolls are tender and translucent and water has evaporated, about 30 to 35 minutes. Stir carefully from time to time to prevent burning.

Add the Garam Masala, cover, and cook for 15 minutes.

Serve with parathas, chapatis, or rice, and a dal.

Cabbage with Potatoes

Serves 4

1 small green cabbage, cored and shredded
4 small or 2 large potatoes, peeled and cubed
1 teaspoon salt
2 tablespoons mustard oil or other vegetable oil
2 cloves garlic, finely sliced
1 teaspoon fenugreek seeds
1 teaspoon coriander seeds (optional)
1 whole dried red chili pepper

In a heavy pan, steam the cabbage and potatoes over low heat until soft. (The cabbage contains enough liquid for steaming without adding water.) Once the vegetables are soft, add ½ teaspoon of the salt.

In a wok, heat the oil over medium heat. Add the garlic and sauté until brown. Mix in the fenugreek seeds, coriander seeds, and chili pepper and roast well. Add the cabbage and potatoes and the remaining ½ teaspoon salt. Stir and simmer until the moisture evaporates.

Serve with chapatis and dal.

Carrots
with Cabbage and Cauliflower

Serves 4

1 tablespoon ghee
½ teaspoon fenugreek seeds
½ teaspoon coriander seeds
3 cloves garlic, finely sliced
1 dried red chili pepper, crushed
4 medium carrots, sliced
½ medium cauliflower, cut into florets
½ green or red cabbage, cored and shredded
1 teaspoon salt
8 whole black peppercorns
4 whole cloves
seeds of 2 black cardamom pods

In a heavy wok, heat the ghee over medium heat. Add the fenugreek seeds, coriander seeds, garlic, and chili pepper. Mix in the vegetables and salt. Tightly cover the wok and cook over low heat until the vegetables are soft, about 35 to 40 minutes.

Remove the lid and increase the heat to high. Cook for 5 minutes to allow liquid to evaporate. (Carrots, cabbage, and cauliflower contain a lot of moisture, and this is meant to be a dry dish.)

Mix in all of the remaining spices and reduce the heat to low for 5 to 10 minutes while the flavors become absorbed.

Serve with any kind of Indian bread—puris, chapatis, or parathas.

Carrots with Peas

Serves 2

½ teaspoon dried pomegranate seeds, soaked in water to cover for 30
    minutes
1 tablespoon ghee
½ teaspoon fenugreek seeds
2 cloves garlic, finely sliced
1 dried red chili pepper, crushed
4 medium carrots, sliced
½ teaspoon salt
1 cup fresh or frozen green peas
1 teaspoon Garam Masala (page 77)

Drain the pomegranate seeds and grind to a paste in a mortar.

In a frying pan, heat the ghee over medium heat. Add the fenugreek seeds, garlic, and chili pepper and cook until the spices are browned. Add the carrots, pomegranate seeds, and salt. Cover tightly and cook over low heat until the ingredients are soft, about 30 to 35 minutes.

Add the peas and sauté for 10 minutes.

Turn off the heat, and allow to stand, covered, for 5 minutes to allow the dish to cool and the flavors to blend.

Add the Garam Masala.

Serve with any kind of Indian bread—puris, chapatis, or parathas.

Cauliflower with Carrots and Peas

Serves 4

1½ tablespoons ghee
1 medium cauliflower, cut into florets
6 medium carrots, grated
3 cloves garlic, finely sliced
1 teaspoon fenugreek seeds
1 whole dried red chili pepper
1 teaspoon salt
4 to 6 bay leaves
1 cinnamon stick (2 inches long)
8 whole black peppercorns
4 whole cloves
seeds of 1 black cardamom pod
1 cup fresh or frozen green peas
1 tablespoon finely grated fresh ginger

In a wok, heat ½ tablespoon of the ghee. Sauté the cauliflower and carrots until lightly browned; set aside.

In a large frying pan or wok, heat the remaining 1 tablespoon ghee over medium heat. Add the garlic, fenugreek seeds, and chili pepper, and sauté for

3 minutes. Add the cauliflower and carrots and stir well. Stir in the salt, bay leaves, cinnamon, peppercorns, cloves, and cardamom. Cover and cook, stirring occasionally, for 10 minutes.

Add the peas and cook over low heat for 15 minutes. Mix in the ginger and turn off the heat.

Serve with rice or any Indian bread—puris, chapatis, or parathas.

Cauliflower with Onions and Potatoes

Serves 4

The vegetables in this recipe are lightly fried, which gives them a special taste and helps them keep their form. Fried vegetables, however, are somewhat heavy to digest.

Basic Soaked Masala:
> ½ cup water
> 1 teaspoon ground turmeric
> 2 teaspoons ground coriander
> 1 teaspoon ground ginger
> 1 tablespoon grated fresh ginger
>
> 2 tablespoons ghee
> 3 cloves garlic, chopped
> 4 medium onions, chopped
> 4 large or 6 small potatoes, peeled and cubed
> 1 medium tomato, quartered
> 1 medium cauliflower, cut into small florets
> 1 cup water
> 1 teaspoon salt

Garam Masala (finely ground):
> 8 whole black peppercorns
> 4 whole cloves
> 4 to 6 bay leaves
> 1 cinnamon stick (2 inches long)
> seeds of 1 black cardamom pod

Combine the basic soaked masala ingredients and let stand for 5 minutes; stir the mixture into a thin paste and set aside.

In a frying pan, heat the ghee over medium heat. Add the garlic and onions and cook until light brown. Mix in the soaked masala and potato, and cook until the ghee surfaces. Add the tomato pieces and cook until they are soft. Add the cauliflower pieces and water and stir until soft, about 15 minutes.

Add salt. Cover, and cook until the ghee surfaces from the vegetables, about 40 to 45 minutes. Turn off the heat, add the garam masala, and let the flavors blend.

Serve with rice or any kind of Indian bread—puris, chapatis, or parathas.

Celery with Potatoes
and Fenugreek Leaves

Serves 2

  1 cup water
  1 celery root (4 inches in diameter), trimmed
  2 large tablespoons dried fenugreek leaves (*methi*), soaked*
  2 tablespoons mustard oil or other vegetable oil
  2 cloves garlic, sliced
  ½ dried red chili pepper, crushed
  1 large potato, peeled and cubed
  ¾ teaspoon salt

In a small pan, bring 1 cup of water to a boil. Add the celery root and cook until soft, about 40 to 45 minutes. Drain and set aside. When cool, peel and dice into 1-inch pieces.

In a wok, heat the oil over medium heat. Add the garlic and chili pepper and sauté for 3 minutes. Add the potato and salt, stir well, cover, and simmer over medium heat for 15 minutes, or until the potatoes are soft.

Add the soaked fenugreek and celery root, and cook for 10 to 15 minutes, until the ghee surfaces again. Remove from the heat. Allow the flavors to blend for about 10 minutes.

Serve with vinegar pickle and puris or chapatis.

*Note: Dried fenugreek leaves should be soaked in water for 5 minutes and then stirred with the fingertips. The dust that settles to the bottom is not good to ingest and should be discarded.

Fennel with Potatoes

Serves 2 to 4

  2 tablespoons ghee
  ¾ teaspoon fenugreek seeds
  1 whole dried red chili pepper
  2 medium fennel bulbs, thinly sliced
  2 medium potatoes, peeled and cubed
  1 teaspoon salt

In a wok, heat the ghee over medium heat. Add the fenugreek seeds and chili pepper and sauté until the pepper turns dark brown. Mix in the fennel, potatoes, and salt. Simmer for 40 to 45 minutes until the vegetables are soft and the liquid evaporates.

Serve with puris, parathas, or chapatis and saunth.

Variation

Other raw vegetables, such as red beets, radishes (red salad or mooli), or turnips, can be used if you don't have enough potatoes. They also should be grated and squeezed of their liquid.

Chinese Mushrooms with Carrots

Serves 4

8 ounces dried Chinese mushrooms, washed and soaked overnight in water to cover

Basic Soaked Masala:
  $\frac{1}{2}$ cup water
  1 teaspoon ground turmeric
  2 teaspoons ground coriander
  1 teaspoon ground cumin

  2 to 3 tablespoons ghee
  1 teaspoon fenugreek seeds
  4 medium onions, chopped
  2 to 3 medium carrots, grated
  1 teaspoon fennel seeds
  1 teaspoon salt
  2 cups plain yogurt
  $\frac{1}{2}$ teaspoon ground cinnamon

Garam Masala (finely ground):
  4 whole cloves
  8 whole black peppercorns
  seeds of 1 black cardamom pod

Drain the mushrooms and retain the soaking liquid. Slice the mushroom caps, discarding the stems. Strain the reserved soaking liquid.

Combine the basic soaked masala ingredients and let stand for 5 minutes; stir mixture into a thin paste and set aside.

In a heavy pan, heat the ghee over medium heat. Stir in fenugreek seeds and roast until browned. Add the onions and sauté until browned. Add the soaked masala and simmer until the ghee surfaces. Stir in carrots, fennel seeds, and salt and mix well. Cover, and simmer until ghee surfaces over the carrots, about 35 to 40 minutes.

Stir in the yogurt and cook for 5 minutes.

Add the mushrooms and soaking liquid and cook until the mushrooms soften and the moisture evaporates. Remove from heat and stir in the cinnamon and garam masala.

Serve with prui, paratha, or any Indian bread, or with rice.

Eggplant Bharta

Serves 2

Bharta is an oven-baked, mashed vegetable.

> 1 medium eggplant, washed
> 1 tablespoon ghee or mustard oil
> 4 medium onions, finely chopped
> 1 teaspoon fenugreek seeds
> 1 teaspoon dried pomegranate seeds, soaked in water to cover for 30
>   minutes*
> 1½ medium cucumbers, peeled and grated
> ½ teaspoon salt
> 1 teaspoon Garam Masala (page 77) (optional)

Preheat the oven to 450 degrees F.

Puncture the eggplant several times with a fork and wrap it in aluminum foil. Bake for 30 to 45 minutes, until the skin is brown and easily penetrated by a fork. Once cooled, peel and mash well with a fork; set aside.

Drain the pomegranate seeds and grind to a paste in a mortar.

In a wok, heat the ghee over medium heat. Add the onions and sauté until the ghee surfaces. Add the fenugreek seeds and cook until dark brown. Add the pomegranate seed paste or substitute. Mix in the eggplant pulp, two-thirds of the grated cucumber, and the salt. Cook over medium heat, stirring frequently, for 10 to 15 minutes, or until all of the liquid evaporates.

Remove from the heat and allow flavors to blend. Add the Garam Masala, if desired. Stir in the remaining cucumber.

Serve with any kind of Indian bread—puris, chapatis, or parathas.

Note: To make this dish less gas-producing and more suitable for aggravated Vata conditions, add a Basic Soaked Masala (page 149) to the sautéed onions and cook until the ghee surfaces.

*Note: Two large tomatoes or 1 teaspoon mango powder can be substituted for the pomegranate seeds.

Eggplant Purée

Serves 4

2 large eggplants, washed
2 to 3 tablespoons ghee
3 cloves garlic, sliced
1 teaspoon fenugreek seeds
1 whole dried red chili pepper
4 to 6 medium onions, chopped
1 teaspoon salt
1 teaspoon dried pomegranate seeds, ground

Preheat the oven to 450 degrees F.

Puncture the eggplant several times with a fork and wrap individually in aluminum foil. Bake for 30 to 45 minutes, or until soft. When cool, remove the skins and mash the pulp into a paste; set aside.

In a heavy wok, heat the ghee over medium heat. Add the garlic and sauté lightly. Add the fenugreek seeds and chili pepper and sauté for a few minutes. Mix in the onions and sauté until their color changes. Complete the recipe in one of the following ways:

Variation 1

Add the eggplant pulp and salt, stir well, and cook for 10 minutes. Remove from the heat and add the pomegranate seeds.

Serve with chaparis, puris, or parathas.

Variation 2 (Additional Ingredients)

Basic Soaked Masala:
$^1/_2$ **cup water**
1 teaspoon ground turmeric
2 teaspoons ground coriander

2 to 3 tablespoons ghee
1 medium tomato, quartered

Combine the basic soaked masala ingredients and let stand for 5 minutes; stir mixture to form a thin paste.

In a frying pan, heat the ghee over medium heat. Add the soaked masala and sauté for 5 minutes. Add the tomato and sauté until the ghee surfaces. Add the eggplant pulp, salt, and pomegranate seeds. Cover and simmer gently for 15 minutes. Remove from the heat.

Serve with any kind of Indian bread—chapatis, puris, or parathas.

Green Beans with Potatoes

Serves 4

3 tablespoons ghee
4 cloves garlic, sliced
1 teaspoon fenugreek seeds
1 dried red chili pepper, crushed
3 medium potatoes, quartered
1 pound green beans, cut diagonally in ⅛-inch slices
1 teaspoon salt

In a wok, heat the ghee over medium heat. Add the garlic, fenugreek seeds, and chili pepper and sauté lightly. Mix in the potatoes, green beans, and salt. Cover and cook until the vegetables are soft, about 40 to 45 minutes. Add water if needed to prevent sticking.

Serve with an Indian bread—chapatis, puris, or parathas.

Green Bell Peppers

with Eggplant and Potatoes

Serves 4 to 6

Basic Soaked Masala:
½ cup water
1 teaspoon ground turmeric
2 teaspoons ground coriander

½ cup finely grated onion
3 tablespoons ghee or mustard oil
3 cloves garlic, sliced
1 teaspoon fenugreek seeds
1 dried red chili pepper, crushed
4 medium or 6 small onions, chopped
1 large tomato, quartered
3 large green bell peppers, thinly sliced
1 medium eggplant, peeled and cubed
3 medium potatoes, scrubbed, peeled, and cubed (new potatoes do not
    need to be peeled)
1 teaspoon salt
1½ teaspoons dried pomegranate seeds, ground

Combine the basic soaked masala ingredients and let stand for 5 minutes; stir into a thin paste. Add the finely grated onion and set aside.

In a wok, heat the ghee over medium heat. Add the garlic and sauté until light brown. Add the fenugreek seeds, chili pepper, and onions, and sauté until the onions change color and the ghee surfaces. Add the soaked masala and cook until the ghee surfaces again. Add the tomato and cook until almost dissolved. Add the pepper, eggplant, potatoes, and salt and cook for 40 to 45 minutes. Add the pomegranate seeds and cook for 3 minutes. Stir, and remove from the heat to allow the flavors to blend.

Serve with chapatis, a raita, and a dal.

Green Peas with Cumin Seeds

Serves 4

1¹/₂ tablespoons ghee
1 teaspoon cumin seeds
1 dried red chili pepper
pinch of asafoetida powder
¹/₂ cup frozen peas, thawed
1 teaspoon salt
6 fresh mint leaves, chopped, or ¹/₈ teaspoon dried

In a wok, heat the ghee over medium heat. Add the cumin, chili pepper, and asafoetida and roast until the cumin seeds turn brown. Add the peas and salt and sauté for 3 to 8 minutes, until the peas are almost soft. Sprinkle on the mint leaves and sauté for 2 minutes.

Serve for breakfast or brunch with 2 to 4 *mathris* (deep-fried salty puris) per person and a sweet fruit cream dessert, for friends with a sweet taste.

Green Peas with Cumin and Potatoes

Serves 4

2 tablespoons ghee
1¹/₂ teaspoons black cumin seeds
1 dried red chili pepper, crushed (optional)
1 cup shelled fresh green peas
4 medium potatoes, scrubbed, peeled, and cubed (new potatoes do not need to be peeled)
2 medium tomatoes, quartered
1 teaspoon salt
¹/₂ cup hot water

In a heavy pan, heat the ghee over medium heat. Add the cumin seeds and chili pepper and roast until the cumin seeds brown lightly. Stir in the peas, potatoes, tomatoes, and salt. Stir in the hot water. Cover and cook until peas and potatoes are soft and well blended, about 40 to 45 minutes.

Serve with chapatis and another vegetable dish.

Green Peas with Potatoes

Serves 2

2 tablespoons ghee or mustard oil
2 cloves garlic, sliced
$^3/_4$ teaspoon fenugreek seeds
$^1/_2$ dried red chili pepper, crushed and roasted
8 ounces fresh, sweet pea pods, washed and cut into small pieces
2 to 3 medium potatoes, scrubbed and cubed

In a wok, heat the ghee over medium heat. Add the garlic, fenugreek seeds, and chili pepper and sauté for 3 minutes. Add the pea pods and potatoes and sauté over low heat for 15 minutes. Stir frequently and carefully.

Serve with parathas or chapatis and dal.

Potatoes with Basil

Serves 4

3 tablespoons mustard oil or other vegetable oil
3 cloves garlic, thinly sliced
1 teaspoon fenugreek seeds
1 dried red chili pepper, crushed
1 large bunch fresh basil, finely chopped
8 medium potatoes, scrubbed and cubed
1 teaspoon salt

In a cast-iron pan, heat the oil over medium heat. Sauté garlic until light brown. Add the fenugreek seeds and chili pepper and sauté until toasted. Add the basil, potatoes, and salt, and stir well. Cover and simmer over low heat until potatoes are soft but still firm, about 35 to 40 minutes.

Serve with any Indian bread—roti, paratha, or puris.

Jackfruit with Onions

Serves 4 to 6

1 pound jackfruit, peeled and cubed
2 to 3 medium onions, chopped
1 teaspoon ground turmeric
2 teaspoons ground coriander
1 teaspoon salt
¹/₂ cup ghee
1 medium tomato, sliced or quartered
4 bay leaves
12 whole black peppercorns
6 whole cloves
seeds of 1¹/₂ black cardamom pods

In a saucepan, combine jackfruit with water to cover. Add two-thirds of the onions, the turmeric, coriander, and salt. Bring to a boil over high heat. Reduce the heat, cover, and simmer until the vegetables are soft, about 45 minutes. Set aside.

In a heavy saucepan, heat the ghee over medium heat. Add the remaining onions and sauté until golden brown. Stir in the tomato, cover, and simmer until soft. Add the jackfruit and onion mixture and cook, uncovered, until about ¹/₃ cup of water remains. Add the bay leaves, peppercorns, cloves, and cardamom and cook for 10 minutes until the dish is dry and the water has evaporated.

Serve with chapatis or puris, and another vegetable.

Variation

For a drier, crispier jackfruit dish, add chick-pea or rice paste to the vegetable when it is almost cooked.

To make chick-pea paste, mix 2 tablespoons chick-pea flour with 1 tablespoon water. For rice paste, soak 2 tablespoons rice flour in 1 tablespoon water for a few minutes. Mix into a paste. Add either of the pastes to the jackfruit and cook over medium heat for 20 minutes, stirring continuously, until the ghee begins to surface.

Leeks with Mixed Vegetables

Serves 2

Basic Soaked Masala:
   1/3 cup water
   1/4 teaspoon ground turmeric
   1/2 teaspoon ground coriander
   1/2 teaspoon ground cumin

   2 tablespoons ghee
   1 medium leek, well washed and sliced into thin rounds
   1 small tomato, quartered
   1 medium zucchini, sliced
   8 ounces chanterelle mushrooms
   1/2 cup grated celery root
   1/2 teaspoon salt
   1 tablespoon finely grated fresh ginger

Combine the basic soaked masala ingredients and let stand for 5 minutes; stir mixture into a thin paste and set aside.

In a heavy saucepan, heat the ghee over medium heat. Sauté the leek until soft and the ghee surfaces. Add the soaked masala and cook for 3 minutes, or until ghee surfaces again.

Add the tomato and cook until dissolved. Stir in the zucchini and cook over low heat for 5 minutes. Add the mushrooms, celery root, and salt, and simmer, stirring constantly, until the liquid evaporates and the ghee surfaces again. Add the ginger. Remove from the heat and allow the flavors to blend.

Serve with buckwheat parathas, any kind of Indian bread, or rice.

Leeks with Potatoes

Serves 4

   2 tablespoons ghee or mustard oil
   1 teaspoon fenugreek seeds
   1 dried red chili pepper, crushed
   3 medium leeks, well washed and sliced into thin rounds
   3 medium potatoes, scrubbed, cubed, and peeled (new potatoes do not
      need to be peeled)
   1 teaspoon salt
   1 medium tomato, sliced or quartered (optional)

In a cast-iron pan or a wok, heat the ghee over medium heat. Add the fenugreek seeds and chili pepper and sauté for 2 to 3 minutes. Mix in the leeks, potatoes, and salt, and cook until soft, about 40 to 45 minutes.

If more liquid is needed, add the tomato, cover, and simmer until dissolved.

Serve with parathas.

Lotus Root with Peas and Potatoes

Serves 4

Basic Soaked Masala:
- 1/2 cup water
- 1 teaspoon ground turmeric
- 2 teaspoons ground coriander

- 2 tablespoons ghee
- 2 medium onions, chopped
- 1 large tomato, quartered
- 2 fresh lotus roots (4 to 6 inches long), washed, scraped, and thinly sliced
- 1 cup fresh or frozen green peas
- 2 medium potatoes, scrubbed, cubed, and peeled
- 1 teaspoon salt

Combine the basic soaked masala ingredients and let stand for 5 minutes; stir mixture into a thin paste and set aside.

In a wok, heat the ghee over medium heat. Add the onions and sauté until golden brown and the ghee surfaces. Add the soaked masala and simmer until ghee surfaces again. Add the tomato and cook until dissolved. Stir in the lotus root, peas, potatoes, and salt and mix well. Cover, and simmer over low heat for 45 minutes, or until soft. For a soupier dish, add a little hot water during the cooking process.

Serve with a dry vegetable dish, kachori, and chapatis.

Dry Okra

Serves 2

- 1 tablespoon ghee or mustard oil
- 2 medium onions, finely chopped
- 1 handful (1/2 cup) dried okra, soaked in water or fresh paneer whey to cover for 2 hours
- 3/4 teaspoon fenugreek seeds
- 1/2 dried red chili pepper, crushed
- 3/4 teaspoon salt

In a wok, heat the ghee over medium heat. Add the onions and sauté lightly for 3 minutes. Mix in all of the remaining ingredients, cover, and simmer over low heat for 30 minutes, or until the okra softens and the liquid evaporates.

Serve with puris, dal, and raita.

Okra with Onions and Garlic

Serves 4

Be sure to wash the okra before cutting, not after; it becomes slimy in water and, like all vegetables, loses minerals if washed after cutting.

Basic Soaked Masala:
    ½ cup water
    1 teaspoon ground turmeric
    2 teaspoons ground coriander

    3 tablespoons ghee
    3 medium onions, chopped
    2 cloves garlic, chopped
    8 ounces small okra, washed and cut lengthwise in 4 pieces
    1 teaspoon salt
    ½ teaspoon mango powder

Combine the basic soaked masala ingredients and let stand for 5 minutes; stir into a thin paste and set aside.

In a heavy pot, heat the ghee over medium heat. Sauté the onions and garlic until golden brown. Add the soaked masala and cook until the ghee surfaces. Stir in the okra, salt, and mango powder. Cover, and cook over low heat for 30 minutes.

Serve with rice or any kind of Indian bread—chapatis, parathas, or puris.

Variations
A red chili pepper can be substituted for the garlic. When served with rice, 2 medium tomatoes can be substituted for the mango powder to provide the sour taste.

Okra with Turnips

Serves 6

Basic Soaked Masala:
    ½ cup water
    1 teaspoon ground turmeric
    2 teaspoons ground coriander

    3 tablespoons ghee
    4 medium onions, sliced
    1½ pounds turnips, washed and thinly sliced
    1 teaspoon salt
    12 ounces small okra, washed and cut lengthwise in 4 pieces
    1 teaspoon mango powder

Combine the basic soaked masala ingredients and let stand for 5 minutes; stir mixture into a thin paste.

In a heavy pot, heat the ghee over medium heat. Add onions and cook until light brown. Stir in the soaked masala and cook over low heat until the ghee surfaces. Add the turnips and cook for 5 minutes. Add the salt and cook for 5 minutes.

Mix in the okra and mango powder, cover, and cook over low heat until the okra is soft and the ghee separates from the vegetables.

Serve with rice or any kind of Indian bread—chapatis, parathas, or puris.

Note: The addition of turnips makes this dish slightly more liquid than most. Okra recipes generally include very little water as it accentuates the "slimy" quality of the vegetable.

Mushrooms with Plantain (Kela)

Serves 4

Basic Soaked Masala:
   1/2 cup water
   1 teaspoon ground turmeric
   2 teaspoons ground coriander
   1 teaspoon ground cumin

   2 tablespoons ghee
   1/2 teaspoon fenugreek seeds
   3 cloves garlic, chopped
   4 medium onions, chopped
   1 tomato, quartered
   1 large plantain, peeled and shredded
   1 teaspoon salt
   1 pound chanterelle (or other) mushrooms, washed, peeled, and sliced

Combine the basic soaked masala ingredients and let stand for 5 minutes; stir mixture into a thin paste and set aside.

In a wok, heat the ghee over high heat. Add the fenugreek seeds, garlic, and onions, and cook until the onions change color and the ghee surfaces.

Add the soaked masala to the wok and cook until the ghee surfaces again. Stir in the tomato and cook until dissolved. Add the plantain and salt and cook, stirring well, for 8 minutes.

Add the mushrooms and cook, uncovered, stirring frequently, for 3 minutes, or until soft and the liquid has evaporated. Remove from the heat and let stand, covered, for 15 minutes.

Serve with chapatis or any other Indian bread.

Mushrooms and Onions

Serves 4

Basic Soaked Masala:
   1/2 cup water
   1 teaspoon ground turmeric
   2 teaspoons ground coriander

   3 tablespoons ghee
   3 medium onions, chopped
   1 teaspoon salt
   1 pound chanterelle (or other) mushrooms, washed, peeled, and sliced
   1 teaspoon Garam Masala (page 77)
   1/4 teaspoon ground nutmeg
   pinch of ground cinnamon

Combine the basic soaked masala ingredients and let stand for 5 minutes; stir into a thin paste.

In a heavy pot, heat the ghee over medium heat. Add the onions and sauté until light brown. Add the soaked masala and salt and cook until the ghee surfaces. Stir in mushrooms, cover, and simmer over low heat for 15 minutes.

If the water from the mushrooms has not evaporated, cook, uncovered, over medium heat until it does.

Add the Garam Masala, nutmeg, and cinnamon and remove from heat. Allow the flavors to blend for 10 to 15 minutes before serving.

Serve with rice or any kind of Indian bread—chapatis, parathas, or puris.

Mushrooms with Soybeans

Serves 4

   2 cups water
   1/2 cup dried soybeans, soaked overnight, rinsed, and drained

Basic Soaked Masala:
   1/2 cup water
   1 teaspoon ground turmeric
   2 teaspoons ground coriander

   3 tablespoons ghee
   4 medium onions, finely chopped
   2 medium tomatoes, quartered, or 2 tablespoons sour cream
   1 pound chanterelle (or other) mushrooms, washed, peeled, and sliced
   1 teaspoon ground ginger
   1 teaspoon salt
   1 tablespoon Garam Masala (page 77)
   1 teaspoon ground cumin
   pinch of ground cinnamon

In a saucepan, bring the water to a boil. Cook the soybeans, covered, for 45 minutes, or until soft; set aside.

Combine the basic soaked masala ingredients and let stand for 5 minutes; stir mixture into a thin paste and set aside.

In a heavy pot, heat the ghee over medium heat. Add the onions and sauté until light brown. Add the soaked masala and cook until the ghee surfaces. Stir in the tomatoes (or sour cream) and mushrooms and cook until soft.

Add the soybeans and cook for 15 minutes. Mix in all of the remaining spices and remove from the heat. Allow the spices to blend for a few minutes before serving.

Serve with rice or any kind of Indian bread—chapatis, parathas, or puris.

Boiled Plantains

Serves 4

3 medium plantains or green bananas
4 medium onions, chopped
2 cloves garlic, sliced

Basic Soaked Masala:
  ½ cup water
  1 teaspoon ground turmeric
  2 teaspoons ground coriander

  1 teaspoon ghee
  1 teaspoon fenugreek seeds
  1 teaspoon salt

In a saucepan, boil enough water to cover the plantains. Cut the plantains, with skins, into small pieces and boil until soft, about 40 to 45 minutes. (Leaving the skins on while cooking helps retain the nutrients.)

In a mortar, mash a handful of the chopped onion and half of the garlic into a paste.

Combine the basic soaked masala ingredients and let stand for 5 minutes; stir mixture into thin paste and set aside.

In a heavy pan, heat the ghee over medium heat. Add the fenugreek seeds and the remaining onions and garlic and sauté until the ghee surfaces. Add the onion and garlic paste, soaked masala, and salt, and simmer until the ghee surfaces again.

Add the plantains and cook over medium heat for 20 minutes.

Serve with any kind of Indian bread—puris, chapatis, or parathas.

Variation

Remove the plantain skin after boiling. Grate the plantain before cooking with the ghee and spices.

Sautéed Plantain

Serves 2

Basic Soaked Masala:
> ½ cup water
> 1 teaspoon ground turmeric
> 2 teaspoons ground coriander
>
> 1 tablespoon ghee
> ¼ tablespoon fenugreek seeds
> 2 medium onions, chopped (optional)
> 3 cloves garlic, sliced
> 1 medium plantain or green banana, peeled and sliced
> 1 teaspoon salt

Combine the basic soaked masala ingredients and let stand for 5 minutes; stir mixture to form a thin paste and set aside.

In a heavy wok or skillet, heat the ghee over medium heat. Add the fenugreek seeds, onions, and garlic, and cook until the ghee surfaces. Mix in the soaked masala and cook until the ghee surfaces again. Add the plantain slices and cook until soft, about 35 to 40 minutes. Add the salt.

Serve with an Indian bread—chapatis, puris, or parathas.

If new potatoes are used in the following recipes, the skins do not need to be removed.

Baked Potatoes
with Raw Condiments (Chokha)

Serves 2

> 3 large potatoes, baked and the pulp mashed by hand
> 1 large onion, finely chopped
> 2 cloves garlic, minced
> 1 to 2 small green bell peppers, minced
> 1 teaspoon salt
> 1 teaspoon ground cumin
> 1 teaspoon mango powder
> 1 teaspoon Special Garam Masala #1 (page 79)
> 1 tablespoon mustard oil

Prepare the potatoes and keep warm.

In a large bowl, combine the onion, garlic, and bell peppers. Add the mashed potatoes while they are as hot as possible, along with all of the remaining ingredients. Mix well. Allow the spices to blend for 15 minutes.

Serve with a dal and chapatis.

Potatoes and Fresh Coriander

Serves 4

4 medium potatoes, scrubbed and boiled until cooked but still firm
2 tablespoons ghee
1 teaspoon cumin seeds
1 dried red chili pepper, crushed
1 teaspoon salt
2 tablespoons chopped fresh coriander leaves

Peel the potatoes and cut into small cubes.

In a heavy pot, heat the ghee over medium heat. Add cumin seeds, chili pepper, potatoes, and salt. Stir well and cook for 10 minutes.

Remove from the heat and stir in the coriander. Cover and allow the flavors to blend for a few minutes.

Serve with puris, or any other Indian bread, or rice.

Potatoes
with Fresh Coriander and Onion

Serves 4

Basic Soaked Masala:
¹/₂ cup water
¹/₂ teaspoon ground turmeric
1 teaspoon ground coriander
1 teaspoon ground cumin

3 tablespoons ghee
5 large onions, chopped
6 medium potatoes, scrubbed and cubed
1 teaspoon salt

Garam Masala (finely ground):
8 whole black peppercorns
4 whole cloves
seeds of 1 black cardamom pod

2 tablespoons chopped fresh coriander leaves

Combine the basic soaked masala ingredients and let stand for 5 minutes; stir mixture into a thin paste and set aside.

In a wok or skillet, heat the ghee over medium heat. Add the onions and sauté until light brown. Add the soaked masala, potatoes, and salt and cook until the ghee surfaces. Add the garam masala and stir-fry until the potatoes are soft and water has completely evaporated. Remove from the heat and sprinkle with the coriander. Cover for 5 minutes to allow flavors to blend.

Serve with puris and parathas.

Potatoes with Onions and Yogurt

Serves 4

Basic Soaked Masala:
- 1/2 cup water
- 1 teaspoon ground turmeric
- 2 teaspoons ground coriander

- 8 small potatoes in their skins, scrubbed
- 4 tablespoons ghee
- 4 large onions, chopped

Garam Masala (whole):
- 8 whole black peppercorns
- 4 whole cloves
- seeds of 1 black cardamom pod
- pinch of ground nutmeg
- 1/4 teaspoon fennel seeds

- 1/2 cup plain yogurt
- 2 cups water
- 1 teaspoon salt
- 4 bay leaves
- 2 cinnamon sticks (each 2 inches long)

Combine the basic soaked masala ingredients and let stand for 5 minutes; stir mixture into a thin paste.

Pierce the potatoes with a fork. In a heavy pan or wok, heat 2 tablespoons of the ghee over medium heat. Add the potatoes and sauté until light brown.

In another pan, heat the remaining 2 tablespoons ghee. Add the onions and sauté until light brown. Stir in the soaked masala and cook until the ghee surfaces. Add the sautéed potatoes, garam masala, yogurt, and water. Simmer until the ghee rises.

Add all of the remaining ingredients, cover, and simmer over medium-low heat for 15 minutes.

Serve with parathas.

Potatoes

Serves 4   ## with Cumin, Fenugreek, and Mint

2 tablespoons ghee
1 teaspoon cumin seeds
2 medium onions, chopped
2 medium tomatoes, quartered
4 to 6 medium potatoes, scrubbed and cubed
1 teaspoon salt
1 tablespoon dried fenugreek leaves (*methi*), soaked*
2 tablespoons finely chopped fresh mint leaves

In a wok, heat the ghee over medium heat. Add the cumin seeds and sauté until brown. Add the onions and sauté until light brown. Add the tomatoes and cook until dissolved. Add the potatoes and salt and stir well. Cover, and simmer for 10 minutes.

Add the fenugreek leaves and mint. Cover and simmer until potatoes are well cooked, about 30 to 35 minutes.

Serve with Indian bread—puris, parathas, or chapatis—and another vegetable dish.

*Note: Dried fenugreek leaves should be soaked in water for 5 minutes and then stirred with the fingertips. The dust that settles to the bottom is not good to ingest and should be discarded.

Pea-Stuffed Potato Patties

Serves 4, two patties per serving

4 large potatoes, scrubbed, baked or boiled
1 teaspoon ajwain seeds
1 teaspoon ground ginger
1 teaspoon Garam Masala (page 77)
1 teaspoon salt
$\frac{1}{2}$ cup fresh or frozen green peas, cooked until soft
$\frac{1}{2}$ cup ghee

Remove the skins and mash the potatoes into a fine paste by hand. Add all of the spices and mix together well.

Mash the green peas into a fine paste.

Place enough of the potato paste into your palm to pat into a small patty, 2 inches in diameter and $\frac{1}{2}$ inch thick. Continue until no potato paste remains.

Place 1 teaspoon of the mashed peas in the center of a patty and cover with a second patty. Firmly seal edges of the patties with your fingertips. Flatten the circles gently with a rolling pin, to make each finished patty about $\frac{1}{2}$ inch thick by 3 inches in diameter.

In a chapati pan, nonstick skillet, or griddle, heat 1 tablespoon of the ghee over low heat. Working in batches, sauté the potato patties, adding ghee as needed after each patty is flipped.

Serve with saunth, chutney, ginger, pickle, and/or a sprinkling of Chat Masala (page 78).

Potato Curry with Onions

Serves 5 to 6

Basic Soaked Masala:
   ¹/₂ cup water
   1 teaspoon ground turmeric
   2 teaspoons ground coriander

   2 tablespoons ghee
   ¹/₂ teaspoon fenugreek seeds
   4 large onions, chopped
   1 large tomato, quartered
   8 medium potatoes, scrubbed and cubed
   1 teaspoon salt

Garam Masala (whole):
   4 bay leaves
   6 whole cloves
   12 whole black peppercorns
   seeds of 1¹/₂ black cardamom pods
   1 cinnamon stick (about 2 inches long)

Combine the basic soaked masala ingredients and let stand for 5 minutes; stir mixture into a thin paste and set aside.

   In a wok, heat the ghee over medium heat. Add the fenugreek seeds and sauté until brown. Add the onions and sauté until golden brown. Add the soaked masala and cook until the ghee surfaces. Add the tomato and cook until dissolved. Add the potatoes and salt and simmer, stirring often, over low heat for 35 to 40 minutes.

   Add the garam masala and cook for 10 minutes, until the potatoes are cooked yet firm. Allow the flavors to blend.

   Serve with puris, parathas, or chapatis.

Potatoes with Bell Peppers and Masala

Serves 4

Basic Soaked Masala:
   ¹/₂ cup water
   1 teaspoon ground turmeric
   2 teaspoons ground coriander

   2 tablespoons mustard oil
   1 large onion, chopped
   1 teaspoon fenugreek seeds
   4 medium potatoes, washed and cubed
   3 medium green bell peppers, chopped
   1 teaspoon salt
   hot water

Combine the soaked masala ingredients and let stand for 5 minutes; stir the mixture into a thin paste and set aside.

In a heavy pan, warm the oil over medium heat. Add the onion and sauté until golden brown and the oil separates. Add the fenugreek seeds and sauté until dark brown. Mix in the soaked masala and simmer until the oil separates again. Stir in the potatoes, bell peppers, and salt. Add enough hot water to cover, and simmer for 45 minutes, or until the potatoes are cooked and the dish is fairly dry.

Serve with Pumpkin with Onions and Garlic (page 167) and parathas or any kind of Indian bread.

Potatoes with Poppy Seeds and Mint

Serves 4

Basic Soaked Masala:
  1/2 cup water
  1 teaspoon ground turmeric
  2 teaspoons ground coriander

  2 tablespoons poppy seeds, well rinsed and soaked overnight in 1 cup
    water
  2 to 3 tablespoons ghee
  2 medium onions, chopped
  1 medium tomato, quartered
  5 large potatoes, scrubbed and cubed
  1 teaspoon salt
  1 handful fresh mint leaves, or 1/2 teaspoon dried

Combine the soaked masala ingredients and let stand for 5 minutes; stir the mixture into a thin paste and set aside.

Drain the poppy seeds and reserve the soaking water.

In a wok, heat the ghee over medium heat. Sauté the onions until light brown and the ghee surfaces. Add the soaked masala and simmer until the ghee surfaces again. Mix in the tomato and cook until dissolved.

Stir in the potatoes and salt and simmer for 3 minutes. Add the poppy seeds and their soaking water, cover, and simmer over medium heat for about 30 minutes, or until potatoes are soft.

Remove from the heat and add the mint. Allow the flavors to blend for 10 minutes.

Serve with chapatis, a raita, and a second vegetable dish.

Potatoes with Dried Fenugreek

Serves 4

2 tablespoons dried fenugreek leaves (*methi*), soaked*
1½ tablespoons mustard oil or ghee
1 clove garlic, chopped
1 dried red chili pepper, crushed
5 medium potatoes, washed, peeled, and cubed
¾ teaspoon salt

Soak the dried fenugreek leaves in 1 cup of water for 5 minutes. In a heavy pan, heat the oil over medium heat. Add garlic and chili pepper and sauté until the garlic is light brown. Add the potatoes and salt and stir-fry for 3 minutes.

Skim the fenugreek leaves floating on the surface of the soaking water. Add the leaves and ½ cup of liquid from top of the soaking water (impurities sink to the bottom) to the potatoes and bring to a boil. Reduce the heat, cover, and simmer, stirring often, until the potatoes are cooked and no water remains, about 15 minutes.

Serve with puris and vinegar pickles with vegetables and fruits.

*Note: Dried fenugreek leaves should be soaked in water for 5 minutes and then stirred with the fingertips. The dust that settles to the bottom is not good to ingest and should be discarded.

Pumpkin with Onions and Garlic

Serves 4

2 tablespoons mustard oil or ghee
2 cloves garlic, sliced
1 teaspoon fenugreek seeds
1 dried red chili pepper, crushed (optional)
2 large onions, chopped
1 medium (2 pounds) pumpkin, peeled and cubed
1 teaspoon salt
1½ teaspoons mango powder, or 1 teaspoon crushed pomegranate
    seeds, or 1 or 2 tomatoes
½ teaspoon jaggery

In a wok, heat the oil over medium heat. Add the garlic and roast until brown. Add the fenugreek seeds and chili pepper and roast for 1 minute. Stir in the onions and sauté until the ghee surfaces. Add the pumpkin and salt, stir well, cover, and simmer over low heat until the pumpkin is completely soft, about 40 to 45 minutes.

For a sour taste, add either mango powder, pomegranate seeds, or tomatoes. Stir in the jaggery and mix well. Uncover and cook, stirring constantly, for a few minutes over medium heat to evaporate excess liquid. Remove from the heat and allow flavors to blend.

Serve with any kind of Indian bread and a vegetable dish.

White Radish with Chopped Greens

Serves 2

³/₄ tablespoon mustard oil or other vegetable oil
1 clove garlic, sliced
¹/₂ teaspoon fenugreek seeds
¹/₂ dried red chili pepper, crushed (optional)
2 medium white radishes (*mooli*), peeled and thinly sliced, the radish
   tops washed and chopped
¹/₂ to ³/₄ teaspoon salt
2 to 3 cups hot water (optional)

In a heavy pan, heat the oil. Add the garlic and sauté until light brown. Add the fenugreek seeds and chili pepper and roast for 3 minutes. Add the radish slices, chopped green tops, and salt. Stir well.

Cover and simmer until soft, about 35 to 40 minutes.

To render into a souplike dish, add the hot water and cook for 8 minutes over medium heat.

Serve with chapatis or any Indian bread and a dry vegetable dish.

Note: Prepared without the garlic, chili pepper, or an excessive amount of oil, this recipe is easy to digest. It is ideal for those suffering from jaundice, as well as for children and the elderly. Select radishes with green, healthy-looking tops. Avoid those whose leaves are pale or have holes in them.

Spinach

with Mushrooms and Potatoes

Serves 4

2 tablespoons ghee
4 cloves garlic, sliced
1 dried red chili pepper, crushed
1 pound fresh spinach, washed and finely chopped
1 pound mushrooms, washed and sliced
4 medium potatoes in their skins, scrubbed and cubed
1 teaspoon salt
2 medium tomatoes, quartered (optional)

In a wok, heat the ghee over medium heat. Add the garlic and sauté for 2 minutes. Add the chili pepper and spinach and toss until the spinach wilts. Add the mushrooms and potatoes and cook until the liquid from the vegetables evaporates, about 30 to 35 minutes. Add the salt and tomatoes, and simmer until the tomatoes dissolve.

Serve with puris or parathas.

Sweet and Sour Pumpkin

Serves 4

¼ cup water
1 medium (2 pounds) pumpkin, peeled and cubed
1 teaspoon salt
1 teaspoon mango powder
2 tablespoons ghee
1 teaspoon fenugreek seeds
1 dried red chili pepper, crushed
½ teaspoon jaggery
2 tablespoons finely chopped fresh basil leaves

In a heavy pan, heat the water and add the pumpkin cubes. Sprinkle with the salt and mango powder, cover, and steam over low heat until soft, about 35 to 40 minutes.

In a wok, heat the ghee over medium heat. Add the fenugreek seeds and chili pepper and roast for 3 minutes. Add the pumpkin (do not drain) and jaggery and mix well. Sauté, stirring frequently, for 5 to 10 minutes, making sure the pumpkin liquid evaporates. The texture of the pumpkin will be very soft, like a pudding.

Add the basil leaves.

Serve with puris or kachoris and a second vegetable or dal dish.

Spinach

with Potatoes and Masala

Serves 4 to 6

1½ pounds fresh spinach, washed
2 large onions, chopped
2 cloves garlic, chopped

Basic Soaked Masala:
    ½ cup water
    1 teaspoon ground turmeric
    2 teaspoons ground coriander

Garam Masala (coarsely ground):
    6 whole cloves
    12 whole black peppercorns
    seeds of 1½ black cardamom pods

    2 to 3 tablespoons mustard oil or other vegetable oil
    4 medium potatoes, scrubbed and cut into 1-inch cubes
    1 teaspoon salt

Steam the spinach until just wilted. Mash in a blender or mortar into a fine paste. Set aside.

Purée half of the onions and garlic in a blender or mortar into a fine paste.

Combine the basic soaked masala ingredients and let stand for 5 minutes; stir mixture into a thin paste.

Prepare the garam masala.

In a clean bowl, combine the onion and garlic paste, the soaked masala, and the garam masala.

In a wok, heat the oil over medium heat. Stir in the remaining chopped onion and garlic and cook until the oil surfaces. Add the onion-masala paste and cook over low heat until the oil surfaces again. Add the spinach paste, potato cubes, and salt and stir well. Cover and simmer over low heat until the potatoes are soft, about 40 to 45 minutes.

To remove excess liquid, uncover and cook, stirring constantly, over high heat for the last few minutes.

Serve with chapatis or puris, tomato saunth, and dal.

Bottlegourd Squash
with Cumin and Chili Pepper
Serves 4

    1 tablespoon ghee
    1 teaspoon black cumin seeds
    1 dried red chili pepper, crushed
    1 medium bottlegourd squash, peeled and cut into 1-inch cubes
    1 teaspoon salt

In a heavy pan, heat the ghee over medium heat. (This type of squash should never be cooked in oil.) Add the cumin and chili pepper and roast for 2 minutes. Stir in the squash, cover, and cook over low heat for 25 minutes. (A cup of water can be added to make a more souplike dish.)

Add the salt and remove the pan from the heat. Allow the spices to blend. Serve with chapatis, puris, or parathas.

Bottlegourd Squash
with Turmeric and Coriander
Serves 4

Basic Soaked Masala:
    ½ cup water
    1 teaspoon ground turmeric
    2 teaspoons ground coriander

    1 tablespoon ghee
    1 medium onion, chopped
    1 medium bottlegourd squash, peeled and cut into 1-inch cubes
    1 teaspoon salt

Combine the basic soaked masala ingredients and let stand for 5 minutes; stir mixture into a thin paste and set aside.

In a heavy pan, heat the ghee over medium heat. Add the onion and sauté until light brown. Add the soaked masala and cook until the ghee surfaces. Stir in the squash. (A cup of water can be added to make a soupier dish.) Cover and simmer over low heat for 40 minutes. Add the salt and remove the pan from the heat. Allow the spices to blend.

Serve with chapatis, puris, or parathas.

Bean Curd

with Tomatoes and Potatoes

Serves 2 to 4

Basic Soaked Masala:
>   ¹/₂ cup water
>   1 teaspoon ground turmeric
>   2 teaspoons ground coriander
>   2 tablespoons ghee
>   2 medium onions, chopped
>   2 medium tomatoes, quartered
>   4 to 6 tablespoons plain yogurt

Garam Masala (whole):
>   8 whole black peppercorns
>   4 whole cloves
>   seeds of 1 black cardamom pod
>   seeds of 1 green cardamom pod
>   4 bay leaves
>   pinch of ground cinnamon

>   2 medium potatoes, scrubbed and cut into 1-inch cubes
>   1 teaspoon salt
>   1 pound bean curd, soaked overnight in water to cover
>   3 cups hot water

Combine the basic soaked masala ingredients and let stand for 5 minutes; stir mixture into a thin paste.

In a heavy pan, heat the ghee over medium heat. Sauté the onions lightly until the ghee surfaces. Add the soaked masala and tomatoes and cook until the ghee surfaces again. Add the yogurt and simmer until the ghee separates.

Stir in the garam masala, potatoes, and salt. Cover, and simmer for 10 to 15 minutes.

Stir in the bean curd and its soaking liquid along with the hot water. Make sure all ingredients are well covered with hot water. Cover and cook over medium-high heat for 40 minutes.

Serve with another vegetable dish and any kind of Indian bread.

Dry Suran (Indian Yam)

with Spices

Serves 2

1 can (16 ounces) suran, or 1 large fresh suran

Basic Soaked Masala:
- 1/2 cup water
- 1 teaspoon ground turmeric
- 2 teaspoons ground coriander

- 1/2 cup mustard oil, to fry yam cubes
- 1 teaspoon fenugreek seeds
- 2 cloves garlic, finely chopped or crushed
- 1 large onion, finely chopped
- 1 medium tomato, quartered
- 1 teaspoon salt

If using fresh suran, preheat the oven to 400 degrees F. Wrap the suran in aluminum foil and bake 1 to 1 1/2 hours, until easily penetrated by a fork. When cool, peel and cut the flesh into small cubes. If using canned suran, cut the pieces into small cubes. Combine the basic soaked masala ingredients and let stand for 5 minutes; stir mixture into a thin paste and set aside.

In a wok, heat the oil over medium heat. Sauté the suran until light brown. Remove from the wok and drain on a paper towel. Set aside.

In the same wok, reserve 1 tablespoon of the mustard oil used for sautéing. Heat the oil over medium heat and cook the fenugreek seeds until brown. Add the garlic and onion and sauté until the onion turns light brown and the oil surfaces. Add the soaked masala and tomato and cook until the oil surfaces again.

Stir in the suran and salt. Cover and simmer over medium heat for 10 minutes, or until the ingredients are well blended.

Serve with chapatis.

Tinda

with Onions, Yogurt, and Soy Yogurt

Serves 4

1 can Punjabi Tinda, strained, or 1 pound fresh tinda

Basic Soaked Masala:
   ¹/₂ cup water
   1 teaspoon ground turmeric
   2 teaspoons ground coriander

   2 tablespoons ghee
   4 large onions, finely chopped
   1 cup plain yogurt
   1 teaspoon salt
   ¹/₂ cup soy yogurt
   ¹/₂ cup water (per person)

Garam Masala (whole):
   2 whole black peppercorns (per person)
   1 whole clove (per person)
   seeds of 1 black cardamom pod (per 4 persons)
   2 cinnamon sticks (each 2 inches long)
   pinch of ground nutmeg
   Dal Masala (page 78)

If using fresh tinda, peel and remove the seeds if they are hard. (If seeds are soft and white, leave them in the vegetable.) Cut into cubes and set aside.

Combine the basic soaked masala ingredients and let stand for 5 minutes; stir mixture into a thin paste and set aside.

In a heavy pot, heat the ghee over medium heat. Add the onions and sauté until light brown. Add the soaked masala and cook until the ghee surfaces. Mix in yogurt and salt and cook until the ghee separates again. Stir in the soy yogurt and cook, uncovered, for 10 minutes.

Add the tinda and water. Simmer, stirring, until one-fourth of the water evaporates. Add the garam masala and boil over medium-low heat for 10 to 15 minutes.

Remove from the heat and allow to stand for 10 minutes.

Sprinkle the Dal Masala over the dish and serve with parathas.

Green Tomatoes
with Potatoes and Onions

Serves 6

Basic Soaked Masala:

    ½ cup water
    1 teaspoon ground turmeric
    2 teaspoons ground coriander

    2 tablespoons ghee
    2 cloves garlic, sliced
    1 teaspoon fenugreek seeds
    4 large onions, chopped
    4 medium green tomatoes, quartered
    6 medium potatoes, scrubbed and cubed
    1 teaspoon salt

Garam Masala (finely ground):

    6 whole black peppercorns
    seeds of 1½ black cardamom pods
    4 bay leaves
    2 cinnamon sticks (each 2½ inches long)
    6 whole cloves

Combine the basic soaked masala ingredients and let stand for 5 minutes; stir mixture into a thin paste and set aside.

In a wok, heat the ghee over medium heat. Add the garlic and fenugreek seeds and sauté for 2 minutes. Add the onions and cook until the ghee surfaces. Add the soaked masala and cook until the ghee surfaces again. Mix in the tomatoes, potatoes, and salt. Cover and cook over medium heat for 35 to 40 minutes. Add the Garam Masala and cook for 15 minutes, or until the potatoes are soft.

Serve with chapatis or puris.

Turnips with Coriander Leaves

Serves 1

    1 medium turnip, peeled and thinly sliced
    ½ cup water
    1 teaspoon packed fresh coriander leaves
    ¼ teaspoon salt

Place all of the ingredients in a medium pan. Cover and simmer over low heat until the turnip is soft, about 35 to 40 minutes. (For a soupier dish, add 1 cup water.)

Serve with a roti.

Turnips with Onions

Serves 4

1 tablespoon ghee
4 medium onions, chopped
1 teaspoon ground turmeric
2 teaspoons ground coriander
8 to 10 small, sweet turnips, peeled and thinly sliced
1 teaspoon salt

In a heavy pan, heat the ghee over medium heat. Add the onions, turmeric, and coriander, and cook until the ghee surfaces. Stir in the turnips and salt. Cover and simmer over low heat for 20 minutes.

Serve with chapatis, parathas, or puris.

Zucchini with Cumin Seeds

Serves 2

1 teaspoon ghee
$\frac{1}{2}$ to 1 teaspoon black cumin seeds
pinch of dried red chili pepper
1 large zucchini, peeled and cubed
$\frac{1}{2}$ teaspoon salt

In a wok, heat the ghee over medium heat. Add the cumin seeds and cook until well-toasted. Stir in the chili pepper, zucchini, and salt. Cover and cook over low heat until the zucchini is soft, about 35 to 40 minutes. (Add hot water to cover for a soupier consistency; this will render an easy-to-digest vegetable even more digestable.)

Serve with a roti.

Chapter Six

PANEER DISHES

  ## Basic Paneer

Serves 2

1 quart fresh whole milk
juice of ½ to 1 lemon, or 3 tablespoons apple cider vinegar
large piece of cheesecloth or clean handkerchief

In a large nonstick saucepan, slowly bring the milk to the boiling point; stir occasionally with a clean spoon to prevent sticking. Reduce the heat to very low and add the lemon juice. Stir slowly and continue cooking until the milk curdles and large lumps of curd form. Add more lemon juice, if necessary. The residual whey will be transparent yellow in color.

Line a deep vessel or colander with the cheesecloth. Set it over another vessel, and pour the curdled milk mixture through the cloth. Tie the corners of the cloth and hang over the sink for 1 hour or more, or until all liquid is drained. At the beginning of the hanging process, squeeze the cheesecloth with your hands to remove excess liquid.

To press the paneer, wrap the curd in cheesecloth and weigh down with a heavy cutting block or iron skillet for 30 minutes.

When all liquid has been expressed, unwrap paneer and cut into ½-inch cubes. Use as directed in any recipe.

Paneer may be crumbled by hand before being added to vegetable dishes, or mashed and used as a filling for breads. It may also be used in sweet dishes. Refrain from using oil as a cooking medium when preparing a paneer dish; ghee is preferred.

Crumbled Paneer

with Soaked Masala

Serves 2

Basic Paneer (see preceding recipe), well drained but not pressed

Basic Soaked Masala:
  $^1/_2$ cup water
  1 teaspoon ground turmeric
  2 teaspoons ground coriander

  $1^1/_2$ tablespoons ghee
  1 large onion, chopped
  1 medium tomato, washed and quartered
  1 teaspoon salt
  2 tablespoons chopped fresh coriander leaves

Squeeze the paneer until it is completely dry.

Combine the basic soaked masala ingredients and let stand for 5 minutes; stir mixture into a thin paste and set aside.

In a heavy pan, heat the ghee over medium heat. Add the onion and sauté until the ghee surfaces. Add the soaked masala and cook until the ghee surfaces again. Mix in tomato and simmer until dissolved.

Crumble the dry paneer and add to the mixture along with the salt. Stir well, cover, and simmer for 10 to 15 minutes, or until paneer turns a yellowish brown.

Mix in the coriander and simmer for 5 minutes more.

Serve with chapatis and a soupy potato dish.

Paneer with Leeks

Serves 2

  $1^1/_2$ tablespoons ghee
  1 to 2 leeks, well washed and sliced into thin rings
  Basic Paneer (page 178), drained but not pressed
  1 teaspoon salt
  1 teaspoon ground cumin
  1 teaspoon Garam Masala (page 77)

In a wok, heat the ghee over medium heat. Add the leeks and sauté carefully over low heat until the leeks soften and glisten with ghee.

Crumble the paneer. Add the paneer and salt and cook, stirring continuously, for 10 minutes.

Remove from heat and stir in the cumin and Garam Masala. Cover and allow the spices to blend for 5 to 10 minutes.

Serve with puris and saunth or tomato salad.

Paneer with Chana Dal

Serves 4 to 6

1 cup black chick peas (*chana dal*), soaked overnight in water to cover
4 cups water
2 batches Basic Paneer (page 178)

Basic Soaked Masala:
   1/2 cup water
   1 teaspoon ground turmeric
   2 teaspoons ground coriander

   3 tablespoons ghee
   4 medium onions, chopped
   1 1/2 teaspoons salt
   1 medium tomato, quartered
   1 tablespoon ground cumin
   1 1/2 teaspoons Garam Masala, freshly ground (see below)

Garam Masala (finely ground):
   6 whole cloves
   1/4 teaspoon black cumin seeds
   1/2 teaspoon white cumin seeds
   1/8 teaspoon ground cinnamon
   1/8 teaspoon ground nutmeg
   seeds of 1 1/2 black cardamom pods
   12 whole black peppercorns

Drain the *chana dal*. In a large pan, bring the water to a boil and add the dal. Cover and cook over medium heat for 45 minutes.

Mash the paneer.

Combine the basic soaked masala ingredients and let stand for 5 minutes; stir mixture into a thin paste and set aside.

Prepare the garam masala.

In a heavy pan, heat the ghee over medium heat. Add the onions and sauté until light brown. Mix in the soaked masala and salt and cook until the ghee surfaces. Add the tomato and cook until dissolved. Mix in mashed paneer, stirring well, and simmer for 10 minutes.

Add the chana dal, stirring well. Cover and cook over medium heat for 35 minutes. When the ghee separates from the paneer, remove from the heat.

Mix in the cumin and 1 1/2 teaspoons of the garam masala. Cover and let stand for 10 minutes, until flavors are absorbed.

Serve with puris or parathas.

Variation

Garbanzo beans, soaked overnight and boiled until soft with 1 teaspoon baking soda, can be used instead of chana dal. Whole kala chana can also be used.

Paneer with Green Beans

Serves 4

Basic Soaked Masala:

    ½ cup water
    1 teaspoon ground turmeric
    2 teaspoons ground coriander
    1 teaspoon ground cumin

    4 tablespoons ghee
    1 teaspoon fenugreek seeds
    1 dried red chili pepper, crushed
    3 cloves garlic, crushed
    4 large onions, chopped
    1 pound green beans, washed and cut into small pieces
    Basic Paneer (page 178), drained but not pressed
    1 teaspoon salt
    4 bay leaves
    2 tablespoons grated fresh ginger
    1 teaspoon Garam Masala, freshly ground (see preceding recipe)

Combine the basic soaked masala ingredients and let stand for 5 minutes; stir mixture into a thin paste and set aside.

In a wok, heat the ghee over medium heat. Add the fenugreek seeds, chili pepper, and garlic and roast for 3 minutes. Add the onions and sauté until golden brown and the ghee surfaces.

Add the soaked masala and simmer until the ghee surfaces again. Add the green beans and cook, stirring frequently, for 15 minutes.

Crumble the paneer and add it, along with the salt and bay leaves; continue cooking until the beans are soft. Add the fresh ginger and simmer for 3 minutes. Remove from heat and stir in 1 teaspoon Garam Masala.

Serve with any Indian bread.

Paneer with Nuts

Serves 4

Basic Soaked Masala:
- 1/2 cup water
- 1 teaspoon ground turmeric
- 2 teaspoons ground coriander
- 1 teaspoon ground cumin

- 4 tablespoons ghee
- 4 medium onions, chopped
- 4 cloves garlic, chopped
- 2 tablespoons grated fresh ginger
- 3 batches Basic Paneer (page 178), drained but not pressed
- 1/4 cup cashews, chopped
- 1/4 cup pine nuts, chopped
- 1/4 cup almonds (soaked overnight and peeled), chopped
- 2 cups fresh green peas, shelled, or 8 ounces frozen peas

Garam Masala (finely ground):
- 1 1/2 teaspoons salt
- 1/4 cup black peppercorns
- 6 whole cloves
- seeds of 1 1/2 black cardamom pods

Combine the basic soaked masala ingredients and let stand for 5 minutes; stir mixture into a thin paste and set aside.

In a wok, heat the ghee over medium heat. Add the onions, garlic, and ginger, and sauté until the ghee surfaces and the ingredients are soft. Add the soaked masala, stir into a paste, and cook until the ghee surfaces again.

Crumble the paneer. Add the paneer and all of the remaining ingredients and stir-fry until ghee surfaces once more, about 25 to 30 minutes.

Serve with parathas.

Paneer with Onions

Serves 4

- 3 tablespoons ghee
- 3 cloves garlic, sliced
- 1 teaspoon fenugreek seeds
- 1 dried red chili pepper, crushed
- 4 large onions
- 2 batches Basic Paneer (page 178), drained but not pressed
- 1 teaspoon salt
- 2 tablespoons freshly grated ginger
- 1 teaspoon ground cumin

Garam Masala (finely ground):
- 8 whole black peppercorns
- 4 whole cloves
- seeds of 1 black cardamom pod

In a wok, heat the ghee over medium heat. Add the garlic and sauté for 2 minutes. Add the fenugreek seeds and chili pepper and roast until brown. Add the onions and sauté until golden brown. Add the paneer and the salt and simmer, stirring occasionally, for 10 minutes.

Stir in the ginger and cumin and simmer for 3 minutes. Remove from the heat, add the garam masala, and stir well. Cover and allow the spices to blend for 5 to 10 minutes.

Serve with chapatis or puris.

Paneer with Red Beets and Peas

Serves 4 to 6

3 tablespoons ghee
4 medium onions, chopped
1 large beet, peeled and finely grated
2 batches Basic Paneer (page 178), drained but not pressed
1 teaspoon salt
1 teaspoon ground cumin
1 cup fresh green peas, shelled, or 8 ounces frozen peas
1½ tablespoons Garam Masala (page 77)

In a wok, heat the ghee over medium heat. Add half of the onions and sauté until golden brown. Stir in the beet, cover, and cook until soft, about 30 to 35 minutes.

Crumble the paneer. Add the paneer and simmer, uncovered, over low heat for 30 minutes.

Add the salt, cumin, and peas. Mix well, and add the remaining onions. Simmer for 15 minutes.

Remove from the heat and add the Garam Masala. Cover and allow the spices to blend for 5 to 10 minutes.

Serve with puris or parathas.

Paneer
with Tomato and Fresh Coriander   Serves 4

Basic Paneer (page 178), drained but not pressed

Basic Soaked Masala:
- 1/2 cup water
- 1 teaspoon ground turmeric
- 1 teaspoon ground coriander
- 1 teaspoon ground cumin

- 1 1/2 tablespoons ghee
- 1 large onion, chopped
- 1 medium tomato, quartered
- 1 teaspoon salt
- 2 teaspoons chopped fresh coriander

Combine the basic soaked masala ingredients and let stand for 5 minutes; stir into a thin paste and set aside.

In a wok, heat the ghee over medium heat. Add the onion and sauté until golden brown and the ghee surfaces. Add the soaked masala and cook until the ghee surfaces again. Mix in the tomato and cook until dissolved.

Crumble the paneer and stir into the mixture. Stir in the salt and simmer for 10 to 15 minutes.

Add the fresh coriander and remove from the heat.

Serve with chapatis and a soupy potato dish.

Fried Paneer with Spinach

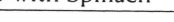

Serves 2 to 4

Basic Soaked Masala:
   ¹/₂ **cup water**
   ¹/₂ **teaspoon turmeric**
   1 teaspoon coriander
   ¹/₂ **teaspoon cumin**

   ¹/₂ **cup ghee**
   Basic Paneer (page 178), pressed and cubed
   1 large onion, chopped
   **1 pound fresh spinach, finely chopped or steamed and puréed to a
      fine paste**
   1 teaspoon salt
   1 large potato, peeled and cubed
   2¹/₂ cups water or whey
   1 teaspoon Garam Masala (see below)
   2 tablespoons grated fresh ginger

Garam Masala (finely ground):
   4 whole cloves
   8 whole black peppercorns
   seeds of 1 black cardamom pod
   pinch of ground cinnamon
   pinch of ground nutmeg

Combine the basic soaked masala ingredients and let stand for 5 minutes; stir into a thin paste and set aside.

In a wok, heat the ghee over medium heat. Add the paneer cubes and lightly fry until brown on all sides. Remove and drain in a colander.

In the same wok, reserve 1 tablespoon of the ghee used for frying and warm over medium heat. Add the onion and sauté until the ghee surfaces. Stir in soaked masala and simmer until the ghee surfaces again. Mix in spinach and salt, cover, and simmer over low heat for 8 minutes.

Add the potato and cook for 10 minutes.

Mix in the fried paneer and stir well. Gradually add the water or whey and 1 teaspoon of the garam masala. Cook slowly until potato is soft, about 30 to 40 minutes.

Remove from the heat and add the grated ginger. Allow the flavors to blend for 10 minutes.

Serve with puris and a *louki* (bottlegourd) or eggplant dish.

Variations

Other vegetables can be used instead of the spinach. If green peas are used, replace the grated ginger with a cinnamon stick.

Chapter Seven

YOGURT DISHES

Plain Yogurt

Makes 2 cups

1 quart fresh whole milk
large piece of cheesecloth or a clean white handkerchief
¼ cup plain yogurt

In a heavy pot, bring the milk to the boiling point, stirring occasionally with a clean spoon to prevent sticking. Remove from the heat and cover with a piece of cheesecloth to keep out impurities. Allow milk to cool until it is a little warmer than body temperature.

Pour the milk into a sterilized glass or stainless-steel container and add the yogurt. Stir thoroughly and cover. (If preferred, pour into individual sterilized glasses.) Set aside in a warm, not hot, undisturbed place, away from light. (The oven can be used if it is set on "warm" with the door left well ajar.) The yogurt will set in about 8 hours.

After it sets, wait 2 to 3 hours before eating. Refrigerate for at least 1 day to stop the action of the yeast on the milk and ensure optimum flavor and texture.

Yogurt with Saffron

Serves 4

3 cups fresh Plain Yogurt (page 186)
large piece of cheesecloth or a clean white handkerchief
1 cup heavy cream, whipped
¹/₂ teaspoon saffron threads, soaked in 2 tablespoons water
5 to 6 tablespoons honey or confectioners' sugar
2 tablespoons slivered pistachio nuts

Pour the yogurt into the cheesecloth and tie the ends together. Hang over the sink for at least 8 hours; the longer it hangs, the thicker the yogurt becomes. (A lined funnel placed over a vessel serves the same purpose.)

When the liquid has thoroughly drained off, mix the thick yogurt with the whipped cream.

Add the saffron mixture, sugar, and most of the pistachios.

Serve in a beautiful bowl, garnished with the remaining pistachios.

Raitas or yogurt salads are an ideal summer food because yogurt is cooling and has a regenerating effect on the system. In winter, yogurt's cooling effect can be balanced with the help of warming spices, such as nutmeg, cinnamon, ginger, or cloves.
A tarka is usually part of a basic raita.

Basic Raita with Tarka

Serves 4

2 cups plain yogurt
pinch of salt

Tarka:
1¹/₂ teaspoons ghee
¹/₂ teaspoon black cumin seeds
1 teaspoon sesame seeds
pinch of asafoetida powder

1 teaspoon dried mint leaves (optional), for serving

In a large bowl, combine the yogurt and salt.

In a ladle or small frying pan, heat the ghee. Add the spices and sauté until well-toasted and fragrant. Add the sizzling Tarka to the yogurt and cover the bowl immediately. Let stand for a few minutes.

Mix ingredients well. Sprinkle with mint leaves to increase the appetizing and digestive value of this dish. Chill the raita well before serving.

Cucumber Raita

Serves 4

1 medium cucumber, peeled and grated
1 cup plain yogurt
pinch of salt
pinch of pepper
Tarka (Basic Raita, page 187)

In a bowl, combine the cucumber, yogurt, salt, and pepper.

Prepare the Tarka and add it to the yogurt mixture. Cover the bowl immediately and let stand for a few minutes. Mix ingredients well.

Chill the raita well before serving.

Carrot and Beetroot Raita

Serves 4

1 cup plain yogurt
pinch of ground cinnamon
pinch of ground cloves
pinch of asafoetida powder
pinch of salt
Tarka (Basic Raita, page 187)
1 medium beet, peeled and grated
1 large carrot, washed and grated

In a mixing bowl, combine the yogurt and spices. Cover the bowl.

Prepare the Tarka and add it to the yogurt mixture. Stir well, and let stand for a few minutes. Add the grated vegetables.

Chill well before serving.

Potato and Tomato Raita

Serves 6

> **6 medium potatoes, scrubbed and boiled until tender**
> **1 cup plain yogurt**
> **pinch of salt**
> **pinch of pepper**
> **Tarka (Basic Raita, page 187)**
> **2 medium tomatoes, washed and cut into small pieces**

Peel and cube the potatoes.

In a mixing bowl, combine the yogurt, salt, and pepper, and cover.

Prepare the Tarka and add it to the yogurt mixture. Cover the bowl immediately and let stand for a few minutes. Stir well.

Wait a few more minutes and add the potatoes and tomatoes.

Chill the raita well before serving.

Onion Raita

Serves 2

> **1 cup plain yogurt**
> **pinch of salt**
> **pinch of pepper**
> **1 large onion, finely chopped**

Tarka:
> **1½ tablespoons ghee**
> **½ teaspoon black cumin seeds**
> **1 teaspoon sesame seeds**
> **1 dried red chili pepper, crushed**
> **pinch of asafoetida powder**

In a mixing bowl, combine the yogurt, salt, and pepper.

In a ladle or small frying pan, heat the ghee. Add the spices and sauté until well-toasted and fragrant. Add the sizzling Tarka to the yogurt and wait for a few minutes.

Stir well, remove the spoon, and let stand for a few more minutes.

Stir in the chopped onion.

Chill the raita before serving.

Boondi Raita

Deep-Fried Chick-pea Drops in Yogurt

 1 cup chick-pea flour
 ½ cup water
 1½ teaspoons salt
 ½ cup ghee or vegetable oil
 1 teaspoon ground cumin
 ¼ teaspoon black pepper

 2 cups plain yogurt, beaten into a thin paste

Tarka:
 1 tablespoon ghee
 1 teaspoon cumin seeds
 2 teaspoons sesame seeds
 1 dried red chili pepper
 ½ teaspoon of asafoetida powder

 tomato slices (optional)

In a mixing bowl, combine the flour with the water and beat until the mixture forms a light paste. If a drop of the paste floats in a bowl of water, the batter is ready. Add ½ teaspoon of the salt.

In a wok, heat the ghee over medium heat.

Using a spatula with medium holes, spoon batter over spatula (1 tablespoon of batter per batch). Jerk the spatula a little, dropping pea-size balls of paste into the ghee. Cook until golden yellow. Drain *boondi* on paper towels and soak in a bowl of warm water for 1 hour. Continue frying until all of the batter is used.

Squeeze the boondi gently to remove the water.

In a bowl, add the cumin, the remaining 1 teaspoon salt, and the pepper to thinned yogurt and mix well. Stir in the boondi.

To make the Tarka, heat the ghee in a ladle or small frying pan. Add the spices and sauté until well-toasted and fragrant. Add the sizzling Tarka to the yogurt. Cover and let stand for a few minutes.

Stir well, and wait a few more minutes. If desired, add the tomato and mix well.

Chill the raita before serving.

Variations

 Moong or urad flour can be used instead of the chick-pea
 flour.

Chapter Eight

SALADS

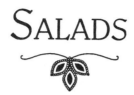

Asparagus Salad

Serves 2 to 4

    1 pound asparagus spears
    1 vegetable bouillon cube, or ½ cup vegetable stock
    ⅛ teaspoon ghee or vegetable oil
    1 tablespoon apple cider vinegar

Marinade:
    2 tablespoons sour cream
    1 teaspoon medium-hot prepared mustard
    1 tablespoon asparagus cooking water
    1 bunch of dill, washed and finely chopped
    ¼ teaspoon salt
    freshly ground black pepper, to taste
    ½ cup watercress or alfalfa sprouts (optional)

Peel asparagus if they are woody. Place asparagus in a heavy pan and add water to cover. Add the bouillon cube or stock, ghee, and vinegar. Cover tightly and bring to a boil. Add the asparagus and reduce the heat to low. Cover and simmer until soft, about 20 minutes. Drain, reserving 1 teaspoon of the cooking water.

    To prepare the marinade, mix sour cream, mustard, asparagus cooking water, dill, and salt and pepper together in a bowl. When asparagus are cool, cut into 1-inch pieces. Toss the asparagus in the marinade. Add the watercress or sprouts, if desired.

Avocado Salad

Serves 4

    1 medium avocado
    1 medium banana
    1 medium orange
    juice of 1 large lemon
    1 teaspoon salt
    1 teaspoon ground coriander
    1 teaspoon ground cumin
    freshly ground pepper, to taste
    roasted sunflower seeds (optional)

Peel the avocado, banana, and orange. Cut the flesh into small pieces.
    Combine the lemon juice with all of the spices. In an attractive bowl, combine all of the ingredients. Sprinkle with sunflower seeds, if desired.

Carrot Salad

Serves 2

Marinade:
    2 tablespoons olive oil
    1 teaspoon fresh lemon juice
    juice of 1 medium orange
    ½ teaspoon salt or sesame salt
    freshly ground black pepper, to taste

    4 medium carrots, grated
    2 medium apples, grated
    alfalfa sprouts (optional)

In a small bowl, combine the oil, lemon juice, orange juice, salt, and pepper.
    Place carrots and apple in a salad bowl and add the marinade. Top with alfalfa sprouts, if desired.

Cucumber Salad

Serves 4

 1 medium cucumber, peeled, seeded, and grated
 2 tablespoons sour cream
 1 teaspoon prepared mustard
 1 bunch fresh dill, washed and finely chopped
 $^1/_4$ teaspoon ground cumin
 $^1/_2$ teaspoon salt
 freshly ground pepper, to taste
 1 clove garlic, pressed (optional)

Press water out of the grated cucumber by hand into a glass; this liquid can be used as a drink or added to vegetable dishes. Place grated cucumber in a small bowl and set aside.

   In a salad bowl, mix the sour cream, mustard, dill, cumin, salt, pepper, and garlic. Add the grated cucumber to the marinade. Set aside for 5 minutes before serving to allow the flavors to blend.

Tomato and Orange Salad

Serves 2

 2 medium tomatoes, washed and cubed
 1 medium orange, peeled and cut into small pieces
 1 medium onion, chopped
 juice of 1 lemon
 $^1/_2$ teaspoon salt
 freshly ground black pepper, to taste
 1 small banana, peeled and chopped (optional)
 10 seedless grapes or raisins (optional)
 $^1/_2$ teaspoon Chat Masala (page 78) (optional)

In a salad bowl, combine the tomato, orange, and onion. Pour on the lemon juice and add the salt and freshly ground pepper. Add optional ingredients, if desired. Set aside for 5 minutes before serving to allow the flavors to blend.

Chapter Nine

CONDIMENTS

CHUTNEY

Chutney is a relish, often sour and spicy, made to accent other dishes. The ingredients should always be fresh and appetizing. Cooked chutneys are often used for special occasions, such as festivals and weddings, while fresh chutneys are used with daily meals. In addition to providing certain vitamins and minerals, chutneys serve to aid digestion and assimilation and also to satisfy the taste buds.

Apple-Avocado-Banana Chutney

Serves 12

5 small tomatoes, peeled and cut into small pieces
juice of 3 limes
3 cloves garlic, minced
½ avocado, the pulp cut into small pieces
1 ripe banana, peeled and cut into small pieces
1 tart green apple, peeled, cored, and cubed
3 handfuls (½ cup) unsweetened coconut flakes
3 small handfuls (¼ cup) raisins
1 tablespoon ground coriander
1 tablespoon salt
1 tablespoon dried pomegranate seeds, finely ground

Combine all of the ingredients in a blender and process slowly until well married. The mixture should have the consistency of a smooth, thick soup.

This chutney is an excellent choice served with pakoras or samosas.

Coriander Chutney

Serves 2 to 3

1 teaspoon packed coriander or mint leaves
1 teaspoon ground dried pomegranate seeds or mango powder
1½ teaspoons salt
1 fresh green chili pepper, ground (optional)

Combine all of the ingredients in a mortar and grind to make a simple chutney. A pinch of this mixture can be taken with every second or third bite of food. It can also be mixed with pulao (rice pilaf) or khichari.

Coriander Chutney
with Apple and Tomato

Serves 6

2 bunches fresh coriander, washed
1 tart green apple, peeled, cored, and chopped
2 medium tomatoes, quartered
2 fresh or dried red chili peppers
1 teaspoon mango powder
1 teaspoon salt

Gradually combine all of the ingredients, in order, in a blender and process to a fine paste.

Serve with pakoras.

Mint Chutney
with Apple and Coconut   Serves 8

2 handfuls fresh mint leaves, washed
2 tart green apples, peeled, cored, and chopped*
1 teaspoon salt
1 fresh or dried red chili pepper
1 cup grated fresh coconut

Gradually combine all of the ingredients, except the coconut, in a blender and process to a fine paste. Add the coconut and blend again.

*Note: If tart apples are not available, 1 teaspoon of mango pow-
          der or the juice of 1 lemon can be substituted.

Mint Chutney
with Pomegranate Seeds   Serves 2 to 3

1 teaspoon dried pomegranate seeds*
1 fresh or dried red chili pepper
1 teaspoon salt
2 handfuls fresh mint leaves, washed

Grind the pomegranate seeds, chili pepper, and salt together in a mortar or grinder. Place mint leaves and ground spices in a blender and blend thoroughly.

*Note: If pomegranate seeds are not available, the juice of half a
          lemon can be substituted.

SAUNTH

Saunth is an appetizing, sweet-and-sour cooked sauce, often served with breads. It can be kept refrigerated for several days in a tightly sealed container. Remove needed amount with a clean, dry spoon but don't bring into contact with water. Saunth has a cleansing effect on the system and is good for the stomach and digestion. It also helps regulate the menstrual cycle.

Saunth with Tamarind

Serves 8

1 cup water
5 tablespoons tamarind pulp
2 cups jaggery
1 cup mixed almonds (soaked overnight and peeled), cashews, and
    pistachios, finely ground
1/2 cup grated fresh coconut
1/4 cup raisins
1/4 cup chopped dates
1 piece (5 inches long) fresh peeled ginger, sliced

Garam Masala (ground):
seeds of 1 black cardamom pod
10 whole black peppercorns
4 whole cloves
1 teaspoon black salt
1 teaspoon white salt
pinch of ground cinnamon
1 tablespoon ground cumin
1 tablespoon ground coriander
2 tablespoons ground ginger

Tarka:
1 tablespoon ghee
1/2 teaspoon black cumin seeds
pinch of asafoetida powder

In a saucepan, bring the water to a boil. Add the tamarind and jaggery and boil until liquid is reduced by half. Remove from the heat and strain.

In a saucepan, combine the strained liquid with the ground nuts, coconut, raisins, dates, and fresh ginger. Cook over medium heat for 40 to 50 minutes.

Remove from heat and stir in the garam masala. Cover and cook for 5 to 8 minutes to allow the spices to blend. Stir in the ground ginger.

To make the tarka, heat the ghee in a ladle or small frying pan. Add the cumin seeds and cook until well-toasted. Add the asafoetida. Add the sizzling tarka to the Saunth and cover immediately. Wait a few minutes, then stir the tarka into the Saunth.

Saunth with Tomatoes

Serves 8 to 10

1 cup water
12 medium tomatoes, washed
5 tablespoons tamarind pulp
2 cups jaggery
1 cup mixed cashews, almonds (soaked overnight and peeled), and
    pistachios, finely ground
1/2 cup grated fresh coconut
1/4 cup raisins
1/4 cup chopped dates
1 piece (5 to 6 inches long) fresh ginger, sliced
2 tablespoons ground ginger

Garam Masala (ground):
    seeds of 1 black cardamom pod
    10 whole black peppercorns
    4 whole cloves
    1 teaspoon black salt
    1 teaspoon white salt
    pinch of ground cinnamon

Tarka:
    1 tablespoon ghee
    1/2 teaspoon black cumin seeds
    pinch of asafoetida powder

In a large pot, bring the water and tomatoes to a boil. Reduce the heat and simmer until the tomatoes are soft, about 5 minutes. Add the tamarind and cook, uncovered, over medium-high heat for 45 minutes to 1 hour. Stir in the jaggery and boil for 10 to 15 minutes, until liquid is reduced by half. Remove from the heat and strain.

In another pan, warm the strained liquid over low heat. Add the ground nuts, coconut, raisins, dates, and fresh ginger. Cook over medium heat for 5 minutes.

Remove from the heat and add the garam masala. Cover and cook for 5 to 8 minutes. Stir in the ground ginger.

To make the tarka, heat the ghee in a ladle or small frying pan. Add the cumin seeds and cook until well-toasted. Add the asafoetida. Add the sizzling tarka to the Saunth and cover immediately. Wait a few minutes, then stir the tarka into the Saunth.

PICKLES

Indian pickles refer to sliced or grated vegetables or fruits. In India, pickles are eaten with breakfast or with a main meal or snack. In some parts of India, breakfast is eaten in the late morning, around 11 A.M. Often it consists of any type of fresh bread, date or lemon pickle, and a cup of spiced tea or chai. Pickles made with lemon juice, like pickled ginger, are often eaten with dal dishes since lemon makes the dal more digestible, especially if the dal is served with a tarka.

Except for the recipes given below, pickles create coughs, colds, and sore throats. These pickles are delicious and can be eaten two to three times a week with the main meal. One should not consume more than 1 tablespoon at a time; 1 teaspoon is usually sufficient. All six tastes—sweet, sour, salty, astringent, bitter, and pungent—are necessary to the body and pickles provide the sour, or sweet and sour, taste. They excite the taste buds and make the mouth produce more digestive juices. Pickles help indigestion, heartburn, and loss of appetite.

Pickles are not good if taken in excess. Too much of the sour taste can thin semen in men and decrease the power of semen retention. (Excess vitamin C has been shown to have a similar effect on semen.) Spiritual aspirants are advised to avoid overuse of sour, bitter, and pungent flavors; only pickled ginger, pickled dates, and pickled lemon prepared without any oil are suitable for them.

Pickled Ginger

---

8 ounces fresh ginger
juice of 4 lemons
$\frac{1}{2}$ teaspoon salt
pinch of black pepper

Clean, peel, and grate the ginger into a bowl. Add the lemon juice, salt, and pepper, and let stand for 30 minutes.

Transfer the mixture to a sealed jar and do not bring into contact with water. Remove needed amounts with a clean, dry spoon.

It will keep refrigerated for about 1 week. Since after this amount of time, it will begin to develop a white fungus, ginger pickles should be made in small quantities.

Variation

Vinegar can be substituted for lemon juice in the above recipe. To make your own vinegar, boil 1 cup of water in a saucepan. Add 2 cups of brown sugar, cover, and cook over medium heat for 45 minutes. Remove from the heat and allow to cool. Pour the contents into a glass jar and seal well. The vinegar will be ready to use in 15 days.

Pickled Lemon

8 small thin-skinned lemons
¹/₂ cup coarse salt or rock salt

Scrub and dry the lemons. Layer the lemons with the salt in a jar. Cover with a tight lid and place in the sun for about 30 days (a windowsill is fine). Shake the jar twice a day so the lemons turn and absorb the salt (lemon will only absorb the amount of salt it needs and leave the rest).

After 2 or 3 days, the lemons will turn brownish and shrink. Continue shaking twice daily until the lemons become soft and turn golden brown, 25 to 30 days in the summer.

These pickled lemons will keep indefinitely without refrigeration, providing the container is well sealed and no extra moisture reaches the mixture. Eventually the mixture will dry up completely.

Serve ¹/₄ lemon per person.

Pickled Lemon with Spices

8 small thin-skinned lemons
1 tablespoon Garam Masala (page 77)
1 teaspoon white salt
1 teaspoon black salt
16 whole black peppercorns
8 whole cloves
seeds of 2 black cardamom pods
1 teaspoon rock sugar candy, ground
1 teaspoon asafoetida powder

Slice each lemon into 8 pieces. Squeeze half the juice from each piece into a small bowl. Add all of the remaining ingredients and mix. Place lemon pieces in a jar and cover with spice and lemon juice mixture. Shake well to distribute the mixture evenly.

Seal the jar and place in the sun for 15 to 20 days. Shake several times a week.

When the skins are soft and have turned a golden brown, the pickles are ready to eat.

Pickled Dates

1 pound pitted dates (20 to 25 dates or a number that will just be
    covered by ¾ cup apple cider vinegar)
¾ cup apple cider vinegar
1½ teaspoons Garam Masala (page 77), ground
15 to 20 whole black peppercorns
8 to 10 whole cloves
seeds of 2 red cardamom pods
pinch of black salt
1 teaspoon white salt
1 teaspoon asafoetida powder
3 to 4 cloves garlic, halved (optional)

Put the dates in a jar and cover with all of the remaining ingredients. Cover tightly and set aside for 3 or 4 hours. Once the dates turn soft and golden, they are ready to eat. (Garlic chunks may be eaten as pickles after 2 weeks.)

    Leftover date pickles can be kept for several months without spoiling, as long as they are kept well sealed in a cool, dry place and no new moisture is introduced. New dates can be added to the pickling mixture. The appearance of a white fungus indicates spoilage.

Pickled Garlic

8 to 10 large cloves garlic, halved
apple cider vinegar or homemade vinegar to cover
¼ teaspoon salt
½ teaspoon asafoetida powder

Place the garlic in a small jar and add vinegar to cover. Add all of the remaining ingredients and cover with a tight-fitting lid. Place in the sun for 15 to 20 days, or until the garlic becomes soft and turns a golden brown.

    Leftover pickles can be kept indefinitely if kept well covered in a cool, dry place. If you have a large jar and use more vinegar, other vegetables (okra, cucumber, zucchini, etc.) or fruits (plums, grapes) can be added.

Pickled Fruits and Vegetables

apple cider vinegar or homemade vinegar, to cover
^{1}/$_2$ teaspoon asafoetida powder
^{1}/$_2$ teaspoon salt
1 cup sliced vegetables and fruits, such as carrots, beets, garlic,
   ginger; seedless grapes, small plums, cherries, apple

In a jar, combine some of the vinegar, the asafoetida, and salt. Add the vegetables and/or fruits and enough more vinegar to cover. Tightly seal the jar. Set the pickles aside for 9 to 14 days.

These pickles can be stored for months, providing the mixture does not come into contact with water. Take out small amounts with a clean, dry spoon. These pickles can be served with vegetable dishes. The remaining vinegar can be used for salad marinades.

Chapter Ten

BREADS

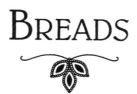

Fresh homemade breads are essential to a balanced Indian meal; they complete the food value of vegetables, salads, and/or dals. They also have many quite tasty and varied forms. The beauty of these breads is that they are prepared fresh, from coarsely ground whole wheat flour, for each meal. Some skill is needed to roll them out in round or triangular shapes, but with a little practice they are easy to prepare. Perfect breads puff up almost to the bursting point during the cooking process, which makes them light and therefore easy to digest.

The breads described in this book are cooked in either a cast-iron skillet or a deep wok. In India, bread is traditionally used as an eating utensil. The thumb and first two fingers of the right hand are used to break pieces off and gracefully scoop food.

TYPES OF BREAD

Recipes for chapatis (griddle-baked flat breads), puris (deep-fried, puffy breads), parathas (griddle-fried whole wheat breads), and mathris (deep-fried salty puris) are all given in this section.

Pappadams are breads, made from bean flour, that become crisp when dry-roasted directly over a flame or when deep fried in oil. They can be purchased ready to cook in Indian food stores. If sattvic foods are preferred, fried pappadams (and pickles) should be avoided.

Indian breads are made without yeast. Whole wheat flour and water are simply kneaded into a soft dough. Salt is not needed when breads are served with spicy dishes.

Any of these breads can be filled with dry vegetables, dal pastes, paneer, or potatoes. (Filling recipes follow the bread recipes.) Finely chopped spinach or onions can also be added to the dough. These breads are at their best when soft, well-cooked, and served hot.

Basic Dough

The following ratio of flour to water will make 3 chapatis, 3 parathas, or 6 puris. The amount of water can be adjusted depending on the fineness of the flour being used; the coarser the flour, the more water is needed.

1½ cups fresh coarsely ground whole wheat flour or chapati flour
⅔ cup water for chapatis or parathas, or ½ cup water for puris

Sift the flour through a medium sieve into a deep bowl. Make a hole in the middle and add the appropriate amount of water; mix well by hand. Rub a little oil or ghee on your hands and knead the dough into a fairly dry, smooth ball. Add flour or water as needed to achieve a workable, elastic consistency. The dough should not stick to the fingers or be dry or hard. With your knuckles, make a few indentations in the dough. Sprinkle on a few drops of water (more if dough is coarse). Cover with an inverted bowl or a clean plastic bag. Allow the dough to stand for 2 to 2½ hours for chapatis, 1½ to 2 hours for parathas, and 1 hour for puris.

Ideally, the dough should be kneaded a second time just before dividing, but it can be used as it is if time does not permit. The softer the dough, the easier the bread is to cook.

CHAPATIS

To Roll Out Dough

Prepare the desired amount of dough from the Basic Dough recipe. After resting for 2 to 2½ hours, knead well. Divide the dough into peach-size balls.

On a lightly floured surface, flatten one ball of dough with your hand. Using a rolling pin, roll out the dough into a thin, round patty, about 5 inches in diameter. Roll from the center, turning patty several times to prevent sticking. Try to make the edges slightly thinner than the center.

Rather than shaping all of the chapatis at one time, cook each one as soon as it is shaped. (If you do shape them all at once, be sure to cover with a damp cloth to prevent drying.)

To Cook

Preheat a cast-iron skillet over medium heat. Remove any excess flour from the chapati by tossing it quickly from one hand to the other. Flip the "stretched" and aerated patty directly into the skillet. When the color changes on the top and bubbles appear, turn it over.

When both sides are done, use kitchen tongs (*chimta*) to remove the chapati from the skillet.

If you have a gas stove, hold the cooked chapati over a medium flame and it will puff up immediately. Turn quickly to flame-bake the other side. Do this several times, taking care that the edges are well cooked. If you have an electric stove, chapatis can be encouraged to puff by pressing them with a clean kitchen towel after the first turn on each side.

Repeat the shaping and cooking process until all chapatis are cooked. To keep chapatis warm as they are cooked, place them in a towel-lined bowl and fold over the sides of the towel. Serve hot, either completely dry or topped with a small amount of ghee or butter.

PARATHAS (TRIANGULAR)

To Roll Out Dough

Prepare Basic Dough and allow to rest for 1½ to 2 hours. To make triangular-shaped parathas, divide the dough into peach-size balls.

With a rolling pin, roll out 1 ball to a circle 5 inches in diameter.

Place a drop of ghee in the middle of the circle and fold the dough in half, to form a crescent or half-moon shape. Gently press the edges closed with your fingertips. Place a drop of ghee in the middle of the crescent, and fold in half again to form a triangle. Seal the edges well.

Dust the paratha with finely sieved whole wheat flour and roll out into a large, flat triangle. Try to make the edges slightly thinner to ensure uniform cooking.

Rather than shaping all the parathas at one time, cook each one as it is shaped.

To Cook

Preheat a cast-iron skillet over medium heat. Add enough ghee to coat the bottom of the pan. Remove any excess flour by tossing the paratha quickly from one hand to the other. Cook over medium heat until the color darkens and bubbles appear on the bottom. Turn and cook until the second side bubbles. Turn again, pressing down on the edges with a spoon. Wherever a bubble erupts, immediately press the area with a spoon or spatula to encourage the air to expand inside the paratha.

Lightly coat the paratha with ghee, turn, and repeat on the other side, coating with ghee and turning. Cook for a minute more and remove the paratha from the skillet. A well-cooked paratha has a golden-reddish-brown color and puffs up like a balloon. Serve immediately or stack in a fresh bread cloth to keep warm until ready to serve.

Variations

For a different taste experience, any of the following ingredients may be added in small amounts to the Basic Dough before cooking parathas:

onions, finely chopped
any chopped green, leafy vegetable, such as spinach or
    fenugreek leaves
salt
pinch of asafoetida powder, or a few drops of liquid asafoetida with
    a few ajwain seeds

PARATHAS (ROUND)

To Roll Out Dough

Prepare Basic Dough and allow to rest for 1½ to 2 hours. Knead well just before dividing the dough. To make round parathas, divide the dough into walnut-size balls; repeat until no dough remains.

Sprinkle 2 balls of dough with a little flour and flatten gently with your palms. Place a drop of ghee (or oil) in center of 1 patty. Press the 2 patties together, with the ghee in the middle. Carefully but firmly seal the edges to form 1 round paratha. With a rolling pin, roll out to a thin, round patty, 6 inches in diameter; turn occasionally to flatten evenly.

Rather than shaping all parathas at once, cook each one as it is shaped.

To Cook

Preheat a cast-iron skillet over medium heat. Add enough ghee to coat the bottom of the pan. Cook the paratha over medium heat until bubbles appear around the edges and throughout the bread, and the bottom has reddish-brown patches. Turn and cook until the second side bubbles. Wherever a bubble erupts, immediately press the area with a spoon or spatula to encourage the air to expand inside the paratha. Turn again and reduce the heat.

With a large spoon, lightly coat the entire surface of the paratha, including the edges, with ghee and massage gently in a clockwise direction. Turn again and apply ghee to the other side. While cooking, press down on the edges occasionally to ensure that the paratha cooks evenly. Cook until both sides are light reddish-brown; a few turnings on each side should suffice.

Serve immediately or stack in a fresh bread cloth to keep warm until ready to serve.

Fillings for Round Parathas

Stuffed parathas and kachoris (stuffed puris) are popular in India. They are served with tea for breakfast, or with a salad at lunch. On picnics, vegetable-stuffed puris are a welcome treat.

The filling must be rather dry, otherwise it will stick to the dough and cause a problem when the dough is rolled out. When raw vegetables are used in a filling, they must be squeezed by hand or through thick cheesecloth or other thick cloth to remove excess water. If boiled or oven-baked vegetables are used, the paratha dough should be made thick and dry. The best fillings are finely mashed so that they do not break through the paratha. If fillings are too moist, they can be dried out in a frying pan.

The following fillings can be used to stuff parathas. To fill, follow the instructions under Round Parathas and place 1 tablespoon of the filling instead of the ghee, in center of the 2 patties. Roll out very carefully so the filling remains inside of the paratha and the dough does not break. Serve hot.

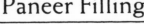

Paneer Filling

Fills 10 to 12 parathas or chapatis

¹/₂ batch Basic Paneer (page 178)
³/₄ teaspoon salt
1 teaspoon ground cumin

Garam Masala (freshly ground):
  4 garlic cloves, minced
  seeds of 2 black cardamom pods
  9 whole black peppercorns

Mash the paneer into a fine paste with your hands. Add all of the spices and mix well.

Stir-Fried Shelled Pea Filling

Fills 10 to 12 parathas

1 tablespoon ghee
1 cup shelled fresh peas
¹/₂ teaspoon salt
2 cloves garlic, minced
2 tablespoons grated fresh ginger
pinch of asafoetida powder
1 teaspoon ground cumin (optional)
1 teaspoon ground coriander (optional)

In a skillet, heat the ghee over medium heat. Cook the peas with a pinch of salt until the mixture softens, about 25 to 30 minutes. Add all of the remaining ingredients, mix well, and mash or blend to a paste.

Variation

Raw shelled peas and/or leafy vegetables or herbs, such as fresh fenugreek leaves, turnips, and very finely chopped cauliflower, can be mixed directly into paratha dough.

Steamed Shelled Pea Filling

Fills 10 to 12 parathas

2 cups shelled fresh peas
¹/₄ cup chick-pea flour, roasted (optional, if needed to make filling dry enough)
¹/₂ teaspoon salt
2 cloves garlic, minced
2 tablespoons grated fresh ginger
pinch of asafoetida powder
1 teaspoon ground cumin (optional)
1 teaspoon ground coriander (optional)

Steam the peas over low heat until soft. Squeeze out any excess water from the peas. Purée them to a paste in a blender. If they are not dry enough, add a little roasted chick-pea flour.

Add all of the remaining ingredients and mix well.

Urad Dal

with Ginger and Dal Masala Filling   Fills 16 parathas

    1 cup urad dal (black gram), cleaned and soaked overnight in water to
        cover
    1 teaspoon salt
    1 teaspoon baking soda
    1 teaspoon ground ginger
    ½ teaspoon asafoetida powder
    1½ to 2 teaspoons fennel seeds, coarsely ground
    1 tablespoon Dal Masala (page 78)

In a saucepan, boil the urad dal, salt, and baking soda in water to cover until
soft, about 25 to 30 minutes. Drain well and mash into a paste.
    Add the remaining ingredients and mix well.
    Serve the filled bread with salad, mint chutney, or saunth.

Chana Dal Filling

                                            Fills 16 parathas

    1 cup whole, peeled chana dal, soaked overnight in water to cover
    1 tablespoon ghee
    3 cloves garlic, minced
    ½ teaspoon asafoetida powder
    1 teaspoon ground cumin
    1 teaspoon salt
    2 tablespoons grated fresh ginger

Drain and rinse the chana dal. Grind into a fine paste in a blender.
    In a skillet, heat the ghee over medium heat. Add the chana dal paste
and cook over low heat until the paste is dry, about 30 to 35 minutes. Add all
of the remaining ingredients and mix well.

Cauliflower (Gobhi) Filling

Fills 6 to 8 parathas

½ medium cauliflower, trimmed into small florets
2 tablespoons ghee
2 cloves garlic, finely chopped
½ medium onion, finely chopped
½ teaspoon fenugreek seeds
pinch of asafoetida powder
1 dried red chili pepper, crushed
¼ teaspoon salt
½ teaspoon ground ginger
1 teaspoon Garam Masala (page 77)

Coarsely grind the cauliflower florets in a blender.

In a wok, heat the ghee over medium heat. Sauté the garlic and onion until golden. Add the fenugreek seeds, asafoetida, and chili pepper. Mix in the cauliflower and salt. Cook over low heat for 10 minutes.

Remove from the heat and stir in the ginger and Garam Masala. Mix well.

Potato Filling

Fills 6 parathas

1 large potato, baked or boiled and cooled
¼ teaspoon salt
½ teaspoon ground cumin
½ teaspoon ground ginger
1 teaspoon ground fenugreek leaves, or 1 teaspoon dried mint leaves

Peel the potato and mash into a fine paste. Add all of the spices and herbs and mix well.

Raw Potato Filling

Fills 8 to 10 parathas

4 medium potatoes, washed, peeled, and grated*
pinch of salt
1 teaspoon Garam Masala (page 77)
1/2 teaspoon salt
1 teaspoon ground ginger
1/3 cup urad flour, roasted

Sprinkle salt over the grated potatoes and set aside in a colander for 15 minutes. Squeeze out the water.

Place the potatoes in a bowl, add the spices and flour and mix into a thick, dry paste.

*Note: Other raw vegetables, such as red beets, radishes (red salad or mooli), or turnips, can be used if you don't have enough potatoes. They also should be grated and squeezed of their liquid.

Mashed Potato Filling

with Onion and Garlic

Fills 8 parathas

4 medium potatoes, boiled or baked and cooled
1 large onion, chopped
1 clove garlic, minced

Masala (finely ground):
1 teaspoon Garam Masala (page 77)
1 teaspoon ground cumin
1 teaspoon ground coriander
1 teaspoon dried pomegranate seeds
pinch of asafoetida powder

Peel the potatoes and mash to a paste.

Grind the onion with the garlic in electric grinder or blender.

In a bowl, combine the potatoes and onion/garlic mixture with the spices and mix well.

Potato Flour Filling

Fills 8 to 10 parathas

1 cup potato flour
¹/₂ cup water
2 tablespoons ghee
¹/₂ teaspoon anise seeds, coarsely ground
1 teaspoon salt
1 teaspoon Garam Masala (page 77)

Make a thin paste from the potato flour and water.

In a saucepan, heat the ghee over medium-low heat. Add the flour paste, anise seeds, and salt and stir into a thick paste. Remove from heat and stir in the Garam Masala.

Serving parathas with yogurt or raita will complement the dryness of the potatoes and make the parathas more digestible.

Turnip Filling
with Onions and Garlic

Fills 4 to 6 parathas

2 medium turnips, washed, peeled, and grated
¹/₂ medium onion, grated
2 tablespoons ghee
¹/₂ teaspoon fenugreek seeds
1 dried red chili pepper, crushed, or 1 fresh red chili pepper, chopped
1 small clove garlic, minced
1 teaspoon salt
pinch of ground nutmeg

Masala (finely ground):
1 teaspoon Dal Masala (page 78)
¹/₂ teaspoon dried pomegranate seeds
pinch of ground coriander

In a frying pan, heat the ghee over medium heat. Add the fenugreek seeds and the chili pepper and roast for 2 to 3 minutes. Add the garlic and sauté until brown.

In a blender, combine the grated turnips and onion. Blend until smooth. Add this mixture to the frying pan and stir over medium heat for 15 to 20 minutes, or until quite dry. Remove from the heat and add the remaining ingredients. Mix well.

Urad Dal Filling

with Garlic and Onions   Fills 8 to 10 parathas

$^1/_2$ cup split urad dal (black gram), washed, soaked overnight in water
  to cover, and drained well
$^1/_2$ teaspoon salt
1 teaspoon Dal Masala (page 78)
$^1/_2$ teaspoon asafoetida powder
1 teaspoon ground ginger
2 cloves garlic, crushed
$^1/_2$ medium onion, chopped and squeezed of liquid

Blend the urad dal in a blender until it forms a thick paste.

In an electric grinder or blender, combine all of the remaining ingredients and grind into a paste. Combine the dal paste with the spices. If the resulting paste is too liquid, heat it in a frying pan over low heat, adding a little urad dal flour until it becomes suitably dry.

Urad Dal Filling

Fills 15 to 20 parathas

1 cup split urad dal (black gram), with or without skins, soaked
  overnight in water to cover and drained well
1 teaspoon ground coriander
1 teaspoon fennel seeds
pinch of asafoetida powder
1 dried red chili pepper
$^3/_4$ to 1 teaspoon salt

Garam Masala (freshly ground):
   4 whole cloves
   8 whole black peppercorns
   seeds of 1 large black cardamom pod

Grind the urad dal to a fine paste in a mortar or blender.

Grind the coriander, fennel seeds, asafoetida, and chili pepper in an electric grinder and add to the dal mixture. Stir in the salt and the finely ground Garam Masala.

In a dry frying pan, cook the mixture over very low heat until the paste is suitably dry.

Varhi (Urad Dal Dumpling) Filling

Fills 6 parathas

Varhis, or badis, are dumplings made with urad dal and Chinese squash. All these dumplings are sun-dried and sold in Indian groceries.

7 pieces lime-sized *varhi*
1 teaspoon fennel seeds, ground
1 tablespoon water

Grind the *varhi* in a mortar or grinder into a fine powder. Add the ground fennel seeds and water and mix into a fine, dry paste. More water can be added, if necessary.

Buckwheat Parathas
with Green Bananas

Make 4 parathas

1 small green banana, or ¹/₂ large plantain
1 cup buckwheat flour
¹/₂ teaspoon salt
2 to 4 tablespoons water

In a saucepan, boil the banana for 40 to 45 minutes, or until soft enough to mash easily, and allow to cool.

Peel and mash the banana in a bowl. Add the buckwheat flour, salt, and 1 tablespoon of water at a time. Using as much water as necessary, mix by hand and knead to obtain an elastic dough.

Roll out the dough and cook according to the (round) Paratha recipe (page 205).

PURIS

Puris are deep-fried breads.

To Roll Out Dough

Prepare the appropriate amount of Basic Dough (page 204) and knead to a firm consistency. Allow the dough to rest for 1 hour. Knead well before dividing the dough into plum-size balls.

With a rolling pin on a lightly oiled rolling board, roll out a ball of dough into a thin, round patty, 2 to 3 inches in diameter. Begin rolling from the middle; with each turn of the patty, add a drop of oil to prevent sticking. Turn the patty often; the edges should be slightly thinner than the center to ensure uniform cooking.

To Fry

Fill a wok or deep skillet one-third full of ghee or vegetable oil. Heat over medium-high heat, but take care not to let the ghee or oil smoke. Test by dropping a tiny piece of dough and submerging it carefully. If it surfaces, the oil is ready for frying.

Gently slide a freshly rolled puri into the wok. As it rises, immediately take a spatula and press it back into the ghee. Position the spatula in the middle of the puri and turn in a clockwise direction. Work the puri toward the edge of the wok making progressively larger circles, until it expands into a "balloon." Turn the puri immediately and submerge it in the ghee; cook until golden brown. Remove with a slotted spoon and drain on paper towels. Cook as many puris at a time as your wok permits. Serve hot.

 # Buckwheat Bread with Potatoes

Serves 2

> 1 medium potato, boiled
> 1 cup buckwheat flour, finely ground
> ½ teaspoon salt
> about 3 tablespoons water

Peel the potato and mash into a fine paste. Add the flour and salt and mix well. Add 1 tablespoon of water at a time, as needed, depending on the fineness of the flour. Knead into a smooth, elastic dough that does not stick to your hands.

Roll out dough like a puri (see above). Cook according to the Paratha recipe (pages 205–206).

This recipe, a good winter bread, provides heat and is also very nourishing. Buckwheat Bread can be served as a simple breakfast with tea, or with vinegar pickle, cumin-flavored peas or potatoes, or any kind of vegetable.

Mathris

Makes 12 to 16, enough to serve 4

Mathris are deep-fried salty puris.

Double batch of Basic Dough (page 204)
$^1/_4$ **teaspoon salt**
1 teaspoon ajwain seeds
1 teaspoon ground ginger
2 tablespoons ghee or vegetable oil plus additional ghee or vegetable oil, for deep frying
$^1/_3$ **cup water**

Prepare a double batch of Basic Dough and work all of the remaining ingredients into it. Knead the dough into a ball and let it stand in a bowl covered with a damp cloth for 2 hours.

Knead again. Lightly moisten a rolling pin with oil. Divide the dough into 12 to 16 walnut-size pieces. Roll out each piece into a flat, thin patty, 2 to 3 inches in diameter. Turn occasionally while rolling. Repeat until all of the dough is rolled out.

In a wok, heat the ghee over medium-high heat. Using a spatula, drop a patty into the ghee and press it to the bottom of the wok, massaging gently. Fry 1 or 2 patties at a time until they rise to the surface and puff up like balloons. Turn each *mathri* over until both sides are evenly browned. Using a spatula, remove from wok and drain on paper towels.

Serve immediately, while hot.

Moong Bread

Serves 2 to 3

with Fresh Green Peppers

1 cup split moong dal, peeled and cleansed
2 cups water
$^1/_2$ **teaspoon salt**
1 to 2 fresh jalapeño peppers
1$^1/_2$ tablespoons Garam Masala (page 77)
1 teaspoon ground ginger
leaves of 1 bunch fresh coriander (if available)
2 tablespoons ghee

In a saucepan, combine the moong dal with the water and salt and simmer until soft, about 35 to 40 minutes.

Drain and grind into a fine paste in a mortar or blender. Add all of the remaining ingredients and mix well.

Place 1 tablespoon of the paste between your palms and shape into a small, flat patty, 2$^1/_2$ to 3 inches in diameter.

In a wok, heat the ghee over medium heat. Cook the moong breads for 5 to 10 minutes on both sides, until golden brown.

Serve with tea and a chutney or saunth.

Chapter Eleven

Desserts and Sweet Fruit Creams

 ## Sweet Balls with Banana

Serves 4 to 6

4 green bananas, ripe bananas, or plantains, boiled in their skins
   (whole) until the pulp is tender
½ cup chick-pea flour
3 to 4 tablespoons jaggery or sucanot
1½ cups water
½ cup ghee
1 tablespoon green cardamom seeds, ground
rose water or kerawater, to sprinkle on top

Peel the boiled bananas and mash thoroughly into a paste.

In a heavy pan, dry-roast the chick-pea flour over low heat for 30 to 40 minutes.

Combine the roasted flour with the banana paste; shape the mixture into 8 to 12 cherry-size balls.

Combine the jaggery and water in a pan and boil for 25 to 30 minutes over medium-high heat until the solution thickens enough to form a thread when poured from a spoon.

In a wok, heat the ghee over medium heat. Deep-fry the banana balls in batches until dark brown on all sides. Place the balls in the sugar solution and allow to cool.

Sprinkle the balls with the ground cardamom and rose water and serve. These balls are tasty, sweet, and an aid to digestion.

Sweet Spiced Bananas

Serves 4 to 6

2 cups mashed banana
³/₄ cup raw sugar
¹/₄ cup water
pinch of saffron
seeds of 6 green cardamom pods, ground

Place the bananas, sugar, and water in a saucepan. Cover and cook over medium heat until the mixture comes to a boil. Remove from the heat and allow to cool.

Place the mixture in serving dishes and add the saffron and cardamom seeds before serving.

Sweet Banana Pakoras

Serves 4 to 6

4 medium-size ripe bananas
¹/₂ cup whole wheat flour
¹/₂ cup jaggery or sucanot
seeds of 4 green cardamom pods, ground
¹/₄ cup ghee

Peel and mash the bananas. Mix in the flour, jaggery, and cardamom. Shape the paste into 16 to 20 walnut-size balls.

In a wok, heat the ghee over medium heat. Add the pakoras in batches and fry, turning constantly to ensure even color, until golden brown. Drain on paper towels and allow to cool.

Chill before serving. These pakoras will keep in the refrigerator for 24 to 36 hours.

Sweet Buckwheat Parathas

Serves 4 to 6

1 large potato, boiled and peeled
2 cups buckwheat flour, sifted
½ cup packed brown sugar, dissolved in ¾ cup water
1 cup mixed cashews, walnuts, raisins, dates, and figs, soaked in
    water to cover for 1 hour
½ cup ghee

Mash the potato and combine with the flour to make a fine paste. Add some of the brown sugar solution. Knead into an elastic dough, adding more sugar solution as needed.

Drain the nuts, raisins, dates, and figs and grind into a paste in a blender.

Shape the dough into 24 walnut-size balls—2 will be used for each patty. Place a small amount of the nut paste between 2 balls and press together. Seal the edges carefully but firmly, forming 1 round ball.

With a rolling pin, roll out into 12 thin patties, each 6 inches in diameter. Turn occasionally to flatten evenly.

Cook in ghee according to the Paratha recipe (page 205–206).

Carrot Bread

Serves 2

2 handfuls whole wheat flour
2 handfuls fine Cream of Wheat
1 tablespoon jaggery or sucanot
2 tablespoons ghee
½ cup powdered coconut
½ cup raisins
1 cup mixed nuts and seeds, such as almonds (soaked overnight and
    peeled), cashews, pistachios, sunflower, cantaloupe, and pumpkin,
    finely ground
2 medium carrots, peeled and shredded
½ cup water or milk

In a large bowl, combine the whole wheat flour and Cream of Wheat. Add all of the remaining ingredients and mix well. Knead the mixture into a dough with an elastic consistency, adding more milk or water if needed. Allow the dough to rest for 2 hours.

Preheat the oven to 175 degrees F.

Place the dough in an oiled loaf pan. Bake for 1 hour, until the top of the bread is brown.

Serve with tea.

Coconut Sweet
with Anise and Cumin

Serves 6 to 8

¼ teaspoon ghee
2 tablespoons ground ginger
1 cup whole wheat flour
¼ cup chick-pea flour
12 cups (3 quarts) water
½ cup jaggery or packed brown sugar
finely grated meat of 1 fresh coconut, or 1½ cups powdered coconut
2 tablespoons anise seeds
2 tablespoons cumin seeds
2 tablespoons ground ginger, roasted in ghee
silver leaves, for garnish

In a hot frying pan, combine the ghee and ground ginger. Roast over medium heat until the ginger turns golden brown, about 25 to 30 minutes.

In another frying pan, dry-roast the whole wheat flour over low heat, stirring constantly. When it emits a nutty aroma (after about 30 to 40 minutes), remove the flour from the pan and repeat the process with the chick-pea flour.

In a heavy pot, bring the water and jaggery to a boil. Cook, uncovered, until the liquid is reduced by half and the liquid thickens, about 40 to 45 minutes. When a small amount of the syrup crystallizes into a hard ball when poured onto a cold surface, add all of the remaining ingredients and mix well.

Pour the mixture into a flat, wide pan, measuring about 18 x 12 inches. When cool, cut into 1-inch squares.

Garnished with silver leaves, this dish is especially good for breast-feeding mothers. Silver leaves soothe and calm the heart.

Cracked Wheat

with Dates, Coconut, and Milk
Serves 2

5 tablespoons cracked wheat
3 cups hot water
10 fresh dates, pitted and sliced
1½ teaspoons jaggery or sucanot
2 tablespoons powdered coconut
seeds of 2 to 3 green cardamom pods, ground
2 cups milk

In a heavy frying pan, dry-roast the cracked wheat over medium-low heat, stirring constantly, for 15 minutes. Add the hot water and cook, stirring occasionally, over medium heat for 30 minutes. Add the dates, cover, and simmer, until the cracked wheat is well cooked and soft, about 20 minutes. Add more water if necessary.

Remove from the heat and stir in the jaggery, coconut powder, and cardamom.

In a separate pan, slowly heat the milk.

Serve the cracked wheat in attractive bowls, topped with the warm milk.

Halva refers to a sweet pudding made with grains, fruits, or vegetables.

Plain Halva

Serves 2

5 tablespoons semolina or chick-pea flour
2 tablespoons ghee
3 cups warm water
5 to 6 tablespoons jaggery or sucanot
1 handful (¼ cup) raisins, washed (optional)
½ cup grated fresh coconut
½ cup almonds (soaked overnight and peeled), cashews, and/or pine nuts, finely ground
seeds of 2 green cardamom pods, freshly ground
pinch of freshly ground black pepper

In a frying pan, dry-roast the flour over medium-low heat, stirring well to prevent burning, until light brown, about 25 to 30 minutes. Add the ghee and stir to form a paste. Slowly stir in the warm water. Cook, stirring frequently, over medium heat for 10 minutes. Add more water if necessary. The consistency of the halva should be very creamy.

Add the jaggery and raisins and stir for a few minutes.

Remove from the heat and add all of the remaining ingredients. Serve warm.

Plantain Halva

Serves 8

2 plantains, green bananas, or not quite ripe bananas
water
1 cup chick-pea flour
1 cup almonds and cashews, soaked overnight in 1¹/₂ cups water
seeds of 8 fresh green cardamom pods, finely ground
¹/₂ cup grated fresh coconut, for serving
jaggery or maple syrup, to taste

In a saucepan, boil enough water to cover the plantains. Add the plantains in their skins (whole) and cook until soft, about 40 to 45 minutes. Drain, peel, and mash into a fine paste.

In a heavy pan, dry-roast the chick-pea flour over low heat until brown and aromatic, about 30 to 35 minutes.

Peel the almonds and grind them, along with the cashews, in a mortar to a fine paste. Remove the paste and set aside.

Add the roasted chick-pea flour, nut paste, ground cardamom seeds, and jaggery or maple syrup to the plantain mixture and mix well. Decorate with the grated coconut.

Serve as a dessert.

Halva with Apple and Paneer

Serves 4

2 tablespoons ghee
1 pound apples, peeled, cored, and finely grated
seeds of 4 green cardamom pods, freshly ground
Basic Paneer (page 178), well drained but not pressed, and crumbled
2 tablespoons rose water
dash of freshly ground black pepper

In a frying pan, heat the ghee over medium heat. Add the apple and carda-mom, and cook until the apple is soft. Mash to a paste, still in the frying pan, over medium heat. Add the paneer and stir constantly, until the ghee surfaces. Allow to cool.

Before serving, sprinkle with rose water and black pepper.

Variation

Pears, peaches, or mangoes may be used instead of apples, if desired. If mango pulp is used, it does not need to be cooked before the paneer is added.

Cooked Sweetened Apple
with Whipped Cream   Serves 4

½ cup water
1 pound apples, peeled, cored, and finely grated
2 cinnamon sticks (each 1 inch long)
½ cup raisins, washed
1 cup sucanot or maple syrup
½ cup powdered coconut
½ cup mixed almonds (soaked overnight and peeled) and pine nuts,
    finely ground
5 tablespoons rose water
whipped cream, for topping (optional)

In a heavy saucepan, bring the water to a simmer. Add the apples and cinnamon sticks and cook over low heat for 35 to 40 minutes. Add the raisins and cook for 5 minutes. Remove from the heat and mix in all of the remaining ingredients. Remove the cinnamon sticks and stir in the rose water.

Serve in an attractive glass bowl, topped with whipped cream, if desired.

Variation (Halva)
Follow the directions above through removing cinnamon sticks. In a frying pan, heat 2 tablespoons of ghee over medium heat. Add the mixture and cook, stirring, until the ghee surfaces. Remove from the heat and allow to cool. Add the rose water and serve. Because of the ghee, this halva is heavier to digest.

Halva with Carrots

Serves 4

1 pound carrots, peeled and finely grated
1/2 cup water
1 tablespoon powdered milk
3 tablespoons ghee
5 tablespoons jaggery or sucanot
1 cup mixed almonds (soaked overnight and peeled), cashews, and
    pine nuts, finely ground
1 cup grated fresh or dried coconut
1/4 cup raisins, washed
seeds of 4 green cardamom pods, freshly ground
silver leaf, for garnish

In a saucepan, cook the carrots in the water, stirring constantly to prevent burning, about 40 minutes. Add the powdered milk and cook until the carrots are very soft.

In a separate pan, heat the ghee over medium heat. Add the cooked carrots, jaggery, nuts, coconut, and raisins and cook for 35 to 40 minutes. Remove from the heat and mix in the ground cardamom seeds.

Cover halva with silver leaf and serve hot, on small plates or in bowls.

Variation

Carrot halva can also be made by boiling finely grated carrots in 2 1/2 quarts of milk, covered, over medium heat until most of milk evaporates. This paste-like halva is then cooked with ghee in a wok.

Potato Halva

Serves 4

4 large potatoes, boiled or baked and cooled
6 to 8 tablespoons ghee
1 cup jaggery or sucanot
1 cup powdered coconut
seeds of 6 green cardamom pods, finely ground

Peel and mash the potatoes.

In a wok, heat the ghee over medium heat. Add the potato paste and sauté well, stirring constantly, until golden brown. Stir in the jaggery and coconut powder and mix well. Remove from the heat.

Put the halva on an attractive plate and serve, garnished with the ground cardamom seeds.

Halva with Mango

Serves 4

½ cup chick-pea flour
½ cup almonds (soaked overnight and peeled), chopped
¼ cup pistachios, chopped
2 tablespoons ghee
2 cups milk
2 to 3 cups fresh mango pulp, mashed
¼ cup jaggery
½ teaspoon ground ginger
8 black peppercorns, freshly ground
¼ cup powdered coconut
3 to 4 tablespoons honey
2 tablespoons green cardamom seeds, ground to a powder

In a frying pan over low heat, dry-roast the chick-pea flour, stirring well to prevent burning, until light brown. Remove and set aside.

In the same pan, dry-roast the chopped nuts for five minutes. Return the flour to the pan and add the ghee. Cook for 5 minutes.

Stir in the milk, mango pulp, and jaggery and cook over low heat until the mixture thickens, about 50 to 60 minutes.

Remove from the heat and stir in the ginger, black pepper, and coconut powder. Set aside to cool.

Add the honey and ground cardamom seeds. Allow to cool before serving.

Variation 1
Omit the milk and substitute Basic Paneer (page 178) made with 1 pint of milk.

Variation 2
Omit the chick-pea flour and milk.

Halva with Noodles

Serves 8

1 teaspoon ghee
4 ounces Chinese wheat flour noodles, dried and eggless
1 cup water
1/2 cup powdered coconut
1/2 cup raisins (or more, to taste)
2 cups milk, boiled and hot
1 cup mixed almonds (soaked overnight and peeled), pistachios,
    cashews, and pine nuts, finely ground
1 1/2 cups jaggery
10 to 12 green cardamom seeds, finely ground

In a frying pan, heat the ghee over medium heat. Sauté the Chinese noodles until light brown.

In a separate pan, boil the water and add the roasted noodles. Cook over medium heat for 20 minutes, or until soft. The water will be absorbed.

Stir in the coconut powder, raisins, and hot milk and cook for 10 minutes.

Remove from the heat and stir in the nuts and jaggery.

Chill. Sprinkle with the ground cardamom seeds before serving.

Halva with Pumpkin

Serves 8

1 medium pumpkin, peeled, seeded, cubed
2 cups water
1 to 1 1/2 cups powdered rock sugar candy
1 cup almonds, soaked, peeled, and finely ground
1 cup cashews, soaked and finely ground
1/2 cup shelled pistachios, soaked and finely ground
1/2 cup powdered coconut
pinch of saffron threads, soaked in 1/4 cup water for 4 hours

Bring 1/2 cup of the water to a boil. Add the pumpkin cubes and cook until soft, about 30 to 40 minutes. Remove from the heat and set aside.

In a large pan, combine the remaining 1 1/2 cups water and rock candy. Boil the mixture until it has the consistency of thin honey when poured from a spoon. Add the cooked pumpkin and mash to combine well. Add the ground nuts and coconut powder. Cook the halva for about 1 hour, or until it has the texture of thick cream of wheat.

Drain the soaked saffron and grind in a mortar. Add the saffron to the halva and stir. Cover for a few minutes and serve warm.

KHEER

Kheer is made from *kshir* (milk). The milk is boiled to evaporate the water, and when enough water evaporates, rice or any other grain is added to make it thick or semi-solid. Nuts, raisins, and seeds with raw sugar are also added to sweeten its taste and enhance its nutritional value. Finally, rose water or green cardamom seeds (whole or crushed) are added to flavor it. Kheer is a good tasting and alkaline sweet dish. It is also a complete food if eaten alone. To avoid using sugar, substitute dates as a sweetener.

It is said that kheer was served to Gautama Buddha by a maiden named Sujata when he was reduced to a skeleton by fasting. After eating the kheer, Gautama realized that an excess of anything is bad, and he formulated the eight-fold path, or "mean path"—*samyak*—and became a realized being.

Kheer is a favorite food of Vaishnavites. It is holy and wholesome. Kheer can be made with squash, cauliflower, zucchini, carrots, and beets to avoid the use of grains. Zucchini kheer is light. If sweetened by dates and enriched by nuts, raisins, and seeds, any kheer is beneficial to all in the seven dhatus.

Serve kheer hot, warm, or cold, as desired. Warm kheer is easier to digest than cold or chilled kheer.

Amaranth Kheer

Serves 2

> 7 pitted dates, chopped
> 1 cup plus 2 tablespoons milk
> 1 tablespoon ghee
> 6 tablespoons puffed amaranth
> 2 tablespoons nuts, finely ground (optional)
> 1 tablespoon shredded fresh coconut (optional)
> seeds of 2 green cardamom pods, finely ground

In a saucepan, boil the dates in the milk until soft, about 30 to 35 minutes.

Mash the dates into the milk with a spoon. Place a sieve over a bowl and pour the date milk through, pressing down on the pulp.

In a frying pan, heat the ghee over medium heat. Add the amaranth and roast, stirring frequently, for a few minutes until slightly brown. Add the date milk and bring to a boil. Reduce the heat and simmer, uncovered, for 10 minutes.

Remove from the heat and add the nuts and coconut, if desired.

Sprinkle with the cardamom just before serving. Amaranth Kheer is not only delicious but also nourishing.

Kheer with Carrots

Serves 4 to 6

> **6 to 8 medium carrots, peeled and grated**
> **1 tablespoon ghee**
> **1 quart milk**
> **2 cups mixed almonds (soaked overnight and peeled), cashews, and pistachios, chopped**
> **1 cup raisins**
> **$\frac{1}{2}$ cup jaggery or sucanot**
> **seeds of 4 to 6 black cardamom pods, ground**

Steam the grated carrots until soft.

In a heavy saucepan, heat the ghee over medium heat. Add the carrots and sauté for 5 minutes.

Add the milk and gently simmer for 5 minutes. Do not allow milk to boil over or burn.

Stir in all of the remaining ingredients and cook over medium heat for 5 minutes.

Serve warm or chilled.

Cauliflower Kheer

Serves 4

> **1 medium cauliflower, washed and cut into florets**
> **$\frac{1}{4}$ cup ghee**
> **1 quart milk**
> **1 to 2 tablespoons jaggery or sucanot, to taste**
> **1 cup powdered coconut**
> **seeds of 6 green cardamom pods, finely ground**

Grate the cauliflower florets.

In a wok, heat the ghee over medium heat. Sauté the grated cauliflower, stirring constantly, until browned.

Meanwhile, in a heavy pan, bring the milk just to the boiling point. Reduce the heat and add the cauliflower. Cover and simmer until the milk is reduced by half, about 45 minutes.

Remove the pan from the heat and stir in the jaggery and coconut powder. Mix well and chill.

Top with the ground cardamom just before serving.

Variation

This sweet can also be made with grated zucchini, potatoes, raw papaya, or pumpkin instead of cauliflower.

Papaya Kheer

Serves 2

1 medium papaya
1½ teaspoons ghee
¼ cup jaggery or sucanot
½ cup nut paste made from almonds (soaked overnight and peeled),
    cashews, and pistachios ground in blender
¼ cup powdered coconut
2 cups milk
seeds of 2 green cardamom pods, finely ground

Peel and seed the papaya. If it is unripe, grate it; if ripe, mash it with a fork.

In a heavy saucepan, heat the ghee over medium heat until hot but not smoking. Add the papaya and cook slowly, stirring constantly, over low heat for 15 to 20 minutes.

Add the jaggery, nut paste, and coconut powder. Cook for 5 minutes over medium-low heat.

Add the milk and bring to a boil. The milk will curdle (this is desirable as it makes the milk more digestible). Reduce the heat again and cook for 20 minutes more, until all ingredients are soft and well blended.

Remove from the heat and sprinkle with the cardamom.

Serve warm or chilled.

Poppy Seed Kheer

Serves 8

1 cup white poppy seeds, soaked overnight in water to cover
1 cup water
1 quart milk
¼ cup sucanot or packed brown sugar

Rinse and drain the poppy seeds. Grind to a fine paste in a mortar.

In a saucepan, bring the water to a boil. Add the poppy seed paste and bring back to a boil. Reduce the heat and add the milk. Simmer, uncovered, until one-fourth of the liquid evaporates and the mixture thickens, about 40 minutes.

Stir in the sucanot. Remove from the heat and serve warm.

Ladoos are sweet balls made of roasted flour or sometimes various nuts and dates. The following recipes provide 2 ladoos per person.

Date Ladoos

Serves 4

2 cups milk
¹/₂ cup heavy cream
1¹/₂ cups mashed dates
1 cup mixed almonds (soaked overnight and peeled), cashews, and walnuts, ground
¹/₄ cup powdered coconut

In a heavy saucepan, heat the milk and cream. Add the dates and bring to the boiling point. Reduce the heat and simmer, uncovered, until the liquid evaporates and a creamy date paste remains, about 45 to 50 minutes.

Remove from the heat and stir in all of the remaining ingredients. Allow to cool.

Divide the paste into 8 equal portions and roll each into a ball, or ladoo. Serve.

Sesame Ladoos

Serves 4

¹/₂ cup sesame seeds
¹/₂ cup jaggery

In a heavy pan, dry-roast the sesame seeds, stirring constantly to roast evenly, until brown. Grind the seeds to an oily paste in a mortar.

In a wok, heat the jaggery, taking care not to burn it. Stir in the sesame paste and mix well. Remove from the heat and allow to cool.

Roll the paste into 8 strawberry-size ladoos.

Chill and serve.

Variation

White poppy seeds can be substituted for the sesame seeds.

Ladoos with Moong Beans

Serves 8

1 cup whole dried moong beans, or 1 cup moong bean flour
1 cup ghee
½ cup jaggery or sucanot
½ cup powdered coconut
1 cup almonds, soaked overnight, peeled, and finely ground
1 cup cashews, finely ground
½ cup shelled pistachios, finely ground
2 tablespoons green cardamom seeds, freshly ground

In a heavy pan, dry-roast the moong beans over medium-low heat for 45 minutes, until the aroma is released and they are light brown. Set aside to cool. Rub the moong beans with a clean cloth to remove the loose skins. Grind the beans into a fine flour in a blender and return the flour to the pan. If store-bought moong bean flour is used, simply dry-roast it in a frying pan over very low heat for 30 to 45 minutes.

Add the ghee to the flour in the pan and cook, stirring constantly, over low heat for 5 minutes. Add the jaggery. Set aside to cool to body temperature.

Stir in all of the remaining ingredients and mix well. Shape into 16 strawberry-size balls and serve.

Rich in protein and vitamins, Ladoos with Moong Beans are ideal for those living in cold climates. Eating 2 Moong Ladoos a day will increase one's strength.

Paneer Ladoos with Saffron

Serves 6

1 teaspoon saffron threads
3 tablespoons milk
1 cup crumbled Basic Paneer (page 178)
2 tablespoons powdered coconut
seeds of 3 black cardamom pods, freshly ground

Grind the saffron in a nonporous mortar, adding 1 tablespoon of milk at a time, and stirring after each addition so threads dissolve completely.

In a separate bowl, mash the crumbled paneer into a fine paste. Stir in all of the remaining ingredients. Pour in the saffron/milk mixture and mix well to make a paste.

Roll the paste into 12 strawberry-size balls.

Chill and serve.

Deep Fried Sesame Ladoos

Serves 4

Ladoos prepared this way are quite heavy and should be reserved for special occasions.

> ¹/₂ cup sesame seeds
> ¹/₂ to ³/₄ cup sucanot
> ¹/₂ cup water
> 1 cup whole wheat flour
> 1 teaspoon ground fennel
> seeds of 2 black cardamom pods, ground
> seeds of 2 green cardamom pods, ground
> ¹/₂ cup ghee, for deep-frying

In a heavy pan, dry-roast the sesame seeds, stirring constantly to roast evenly, until brown. Grind the seeds with the sucanot to an oily paste in a mortar.

Place the paste in a large bowl and mix in the water, flour, and spices. Knead very well, to a dough-like consistency.

Roll the dough into strawberry-size ladoos.

In a wok, heat the ghee over medium-high heat. Deep-fry the ladoos, stirring constantly, until browned evenly all over. Drain on paper towels.

Chill and serve.

Ladoos

Serves 4   with Cream of Wheat and Wheat Germ

> ¹/₂ cup ghee
> 1 cup Cream of Wheat
> 1 cup wheat germ
> ¹/₂ cup sucanot or jaggery
> ¹/₂ cup powdered coconut
> 1 cup almonds, soaked overnight and peeled
> 1 cup cashews
> 1 cup shelled pistachios
> seeds of 2 green cardamom pods, finely ground
> 8 to 10 black peppercorns, freshly ground

In a wok, heat the ghee over medium heat. Add the Cream of Wheat and wheat germ and cook, stirring constantly, until golden brown, about 30 to 35 minutes.

Add the jaggery and mix well; remove from heat.

With an electric grinder or blender, process the powdered coconut and all of the nuts into a paste. Add the nut paste to the wheat/jaggery mixture. Stir well and add the ground cardamom and black pepper.

Using 1 tablespoon of the paste for each, roll the dough into small balls.

Chill and serve. This type of ladoo balances the three humors. Wheat germ, rich in vitamin E, helps cure constipation and is good for the skin.

Chick-pea Flour Ladoos

Serves 4 to 6

1 cup chick-pea flour
¼ cup ghee
½ cup jaggery or sucanot
½ cup nut paste, made from almonds (soaked overnight and peeled),
**   cashews, and pistachios ground in a blender**
seeds of 6 to 8 green cardamom pods, crushed

In a heavy frying pan or wok, dry-roast the chick-pea flour over low heat until it turns golden brown and releases its aroma, about 30 to 40 minutes.

Add the ghee and cook, stirring, for 5 to 10 minutes, or until the chick-pea flour absorbs the ghee and becomes crisp.

Add the jaggery and nut paste. Stir well and cook for 5 to 10 minutes. Remove from the heat and stir in the crushed cardamom.

After the mixture cools a little, shape the paste into walnut-size balls. Serve room temperature or chilled.

Rabri

with Pistachios and Cardamom   Serves 2

Rabri is sweetened milk that has been reduced.

1 quart fresh milk
3 tablespoons jaggery or sucanot
½ cup shelled pistachios, finely ground
seeds of 10 green cardamom pods, freshly ground

In a cast-iron skillet or wok, heat the milk slowly over medium heat until reduced to half of its original amount. Stir frequently to prevent burning. When it acquires a cream-like consistency, add the jaggery and remove from the heat. Mix in the pistachios and cardamom seeds. Return to low heat, cover, and cook until reduced again by half and the consistency of thick honey, about 1¼ hours.

Serve as a dressing over mangoes or other fruits, or as a topping for fruit salads.

Meusli

Serves 4

½ cup wheat germ, or ½ cup coarsely ground whole wheat flour,
    sifted
2 cups warm water
2 cups milk
4 to 7 dates, pitted and sliced
3 tablespoons jaggery or sucanot
1 tablespoon ghee
½ cup raisins, washed
½ cup coconut flakes
½ cup mixed almonds (soaked overnight and peeled), cashews, and
    pine nuts, finely chopped
thinly sliced seasonal fruit (optional)

In a heavy pan, dry-roast the wheat germ or flour over low heat, stirring carefully to prevent burning, until the wheat germ emits a nut-like aroma, about 15 to 20 minutes.

Add the warm water, milk, and dates (add more warm water if necessary for a honey-like consistency). Cook over low heat until the mixture swells and softens, about 15 minutes.

Add the jaggery, ghee, and raisins. Stir well and remove pan from the heat. Stir in the coconut and nuts. Serve with fruit, if desired.

Variation

Use equal amounts of wheat germ and rolled oats. At the end of cooking, 1 tablespoon of roasted linseeds or yeast flakes can be added.

Sweet Potato
with Milk and Coconut

Serves 2 to 4

1 large sweet potato
finely shredded meat of 1 fresh coconut
2 to 4 teaspoons packed brown sugar
seeds of 2 to 4 green cardamom pods, freshly ground
½ cup fresh milk, warmed

Preheat the oven to 400 degrees F.

Puncture the potato several times with a fork. Bake for 40 minutes, or until soft. Alternately, boil the sweet potato.

When cooled, peel the potato and place in a bowl. Mash into a paste and add the shredded coconut, brown sugar, and cardamom. Mix very well and gradually add the warm milk.

Chill before serving.

Sweet Puris with Nut Filling

Serves 4

1 1/2 cups whole wheat flour
2 tablespoons plus 1/2 cup ghee
1 cup mixed nuts and seeds, such as soaked and peeled almonds,
**   cashews, shelled pistachios, sunflower, cantaloupe, and pumpkin**
1/2 cup packed brown sugar dissolved in 1 cup water
about 2 cups cold milk
1 teaspoon rose water

Mix the whole wheat flour with 2 tablespoons of the ghee.

Grind the nuts and seeds into an oily paste in a mortar; set aside.

In a medium bowl, combine the flour mixture and sugar solution; mix well to form a dough. Let rest for 30 to 40 minutes.

Shape the dough into 16 walnut-size balls—2 for each final patty. Place a small amount of the nut paste between 2 balls of dough and press together. Seal the edges carefully but firmly, forming 1 ball.

Using a rolling pin, roll out 8 thin patties, each about 6 inches in diameter. Turn occasionally to flatten evenly.

In a wok, heat the remaining 1/2 cup ghee over medium-high heat. When hot, add the puris and fry on both sides until well cooked and puffy. Remove and drain in a paper-lined bowl; let cool to room temperature.

Remove the paper and pour enough cold milk in bowl to cover the puris. Set aside to soak for 3 to 6 hours at room temperature.

Add the rose water and serve.

Sweet Whole Wheat Flour Balls

Serves 4 to 6

2 cups whole wheat flour
¹/₂ cup sesame seeds
¹/₂ cup cashews
¹/₄ cup ghee
¹/₂ cup jaggery or sucanot
¹/₂ cup raisins
seeds of 4 to 6 green cardamom pods, finely ground
¹/₂ cup powdered coconut

In a frying pan, dry-roast the whole wheat flour over low heat, stirring constantly, until the flour changes color and emits a nutty aroma, about 30 to 40 minutes. Remove from the pan.

In the same pan, dry-roast the sesame seeds and cashews until golden brown. Mash the seeds and nuts into a paste in a mortar.

Return the roasted flour and roasted nut/seed mixture to the frying pan over low heat. Add the ghee and cook for 2 to 3 minutes, or until the mixture is uniform. Add the jaggery and stir until blended. Add the raisins and ground cardamom and mix well.

Shape the dough into 8 to 12 small balls. Roll in the coconut powder while still warm.

Serve to lovers of sweets.

SWEET FRUIT CREAMS

Banana Cream with Rose Petals

Serves 4

2 large ripe bananas
1 tablespoon honey
¼ cup heavy cream
4 teaspoons rose petal jam (*gulkand*)

Mash the bananas with the honey until creamy.

In a large bowl, whip the sweet cream until stiff. Fold in the mashed banana and mix well.

Chill and serve in small dessert dishes, topping each portion with 1 teaspoon of the rose petal jam.

Date Sweet Cream

Serves 4

18 fresh dates, pitted and chopped
1 teaspoon honey
1 cup heavy cream
seeds of 4 fresh green cardamom pods, finely ground

Grind the dates to a fine paste in a mortar or blender.

In a bowl, combine the honey and heavy cream; whip until just thickened. Add the dates and ground cardamom and stir well.

Chill and serve in attractive bowls.

Papaya Sweet Cream

Serves 2

1 medium-size ripe papaya, peeled, seeded, and coarsely chopped
1 tablespoon maple syrup
1 tablespoon rose water
1 cup heavy cream

In a blender, combine the papaya, maple syrup, and rose water. Add the heavy cream to the blender, and whip for a few seconds, until just thickened.

Serve in dessert bowls as is, or refrigerate for 1 hour if a thicker consistency is desired.

Mango Sweet Cream

Serves 2

1 ripe mango
1 cup heavy cream
1 tablespoon maple syrup
1 tablespoon rose water
2 tablespoons rose petal jam (*gulkand*) (optional)

Place the mango in the refrigerator or in cold water for at least 30 minutes before using.

In a bowl, whip the cream until just thickened. Cover and refrigerate.

Cut the mango lengthwise in half, slicing around the pit. With a tablespoon, scrape the pulp from each half and from the pit.

Blend the mango pulp, maple syrup, and rose water in a blender. Fold in the whipped cream. Serve in dessert bowls, topping each dish with 1 teaspoon of the rose petal jam, if desired.

Peach-Banana-Apple Sweet Cream

Serves 4

3 medium very ripe peaches
2 medium apples
2 medium bananas
1/2 cup raisins, soaked in water for 45 minutes and drained, or 1/2 cup chopped pitted dates
1/4 cup powdered coconut
1 tablespoon honey or maple syrup
1 cup heavy cream
seeds of 2 green cardamom pods, finely ground

Peel and pit or core the peaches and apples. Cut the peaches and bananas into small pieces, and grate the apples.

In a large bowl, combine the fruits, raisins, coconut powder, and honey.

In a separate bowl, whip the cream until just thickened. Sprinkle the cream with the ground cardamom. Fold the cream into the fruit mixture.

Chill and serve in dessert bowls.

Strawberry-Banana Sweet Cream

Serves 4

2 cups fresh strawberries, washed and dried
2 medium bananas, mashed
$\frac{1}{4}$ cup coconut powder
1 to 2 tablespoons honey or maple syrup
1 cup heavy cream
seeds of 2 green cardamom pods, finely ground

Stem and thinly slice the strawberries. Stir in the mashed bananas, coconut powder, and honey.

In a separate bowl, whip the cream until just thickened. Sprinkle the cream with the ground cardamom. Fold into the fruit mixture.

Chill and serve in dessert bowls.

Chapter Twelve

BEVERAGES

Many of the recipes that follow call for water. Pure spring water is ideal for drinking and cooking. Those who inhabit modern metropolitan areas, however, have access only to whatever type of water flows from their taps. As a precautionary measure, ordinary tap water can be boiled for 5 to 10 minutes, then cooled to body temperature. Boiling removes enough of certain additives, such as chlorine, in their gaseous form so we cannot taste them. Aerate boiled water before drinking by pouring it carefully from one glass to another. Boiling water causes it to lose negative ions through evaporation.

In addition to the recipes listed below, the whey from fresh paneer is very nutritious, although it cannot be stored. A teaspoon of honey can be added to each 8-ounce glass of paneer whey. Red beet juice also provides nourishment and energy. It is a tonic for anemic and weak people.

The small blackish cardamom seeds used in the beverages are from green cardamom pods. Four green pods yield about ¼ teaspoon of seeds.

The beverages that follow can be drunk alone or after eating.

Dal Water

Providing the dal has been thoroughly cleaned beforehand, the water used to soak dal can be drunk. It can be served to invalids, infants, and weak people who may be unable to ingest dal itself. When the water is to be drunk, do not use baking soda when cooking the dal.

Water from cooked chana dal beans, which is especially rich in protein and iron, can be served as a drink by adding 2 teaspoons of honey per glass.

Banana Drink

Serves 4 to 6

12 bananas, peeled and thinly sliced
2 tablespoons jaggery
water to cover
7 saffron threads, soaked in enough water to moisten and then ground
seeds of 4 to 6 cardamom pods, freshly ground

Combine the bananas and jaggery in a heavy saucepan. Add the water and tightly cover. Slowly bring to a boil; immediately turn off the heat. Refrigerate for ½ hour.

Before serving, stir in the saffron liquid and ground cardamom.

Magic Drink

Serves 4

Magic Drink is a good source of proteins and vitamins.

½ cup honeydew melon seeds, dried and peeled*
½ cup pumpkin seeds
2 tablespoons white poppy seeds
2 tablespoons anise seeds
1 quart milk
2 tablespoons almond oil or ghee
1 tablespoon jaggery
freshly ground black pepper, to taste

Soak the honeydew melon and pumpkin seeds in water to cover overnight.

The next morning, drain the seeds and grind, along with the poppy and anise seeds, in a small amount of the milk in a mortar or electric grinder.

In a heavy pan, heat the oil over low heat. Add the liquid nut paste and roast for 1 minute, stirring well to avoid burning. Add the remaining milk and bring just to a boil. Remove from the heat as soon as bubbles begin to rise.

Set aside to cool for 5 minutes. Stir in the jaggery.

Pour into glasses and sprinkle each glass with black pepper to taste.

*Note: If honeydew melon seeds are not available, ½ cup sunflower seeds and 1 cup of mixed nuts—almonds, cashews, and pine nuts—soaked overnight can be used. (Peel almonds before using.)

Mango Shake

Serves 4

9 saffron threads
1 quart plus 3 tablespoons milk
1 large ripe mango
1 cup heavy cream
4 teaspoons honey
rosewater, or the freshly ground seeds of 8 green cardamom pods, for
serving

Grind the saffron threads in a mortar with 3 tablespoons of the milk.

Peel the mango and remove the seed. Mash the pulp in a blender. Add the remaining 1 quart milk, the cream, and saffron thread liquid. Blend well.

To each glass, add 1 teaspoon of honey and 8 to 10 drops of rosewater or some of the ground cardamom.

Spiced Milk

Serves 1

1 cup milk
1 whole clove
seeds of 1 green cardamom pod, freshly ground
½ teaspoon jaggery or sucanot
sliver of 1 vanilla bean

Heat the milk until it boils; remove from the heat as soon as bubbles begin to rise. Stir in all of the remaining ingredients. Cover and let steep for 5 to 10 minutes.

Strain into a glass and serve.

Cardamom Milk

Serves 1

1 cup milk
½ to 1 teaspoon jaggery or sucanot
seeds of 1 green cardamom pod, freshly ground

Heat the milk until it boils; remove from the heat as soon as bubbles begin to rise. Stir in the jaggery and cardamom. Cover and let steep for 5 to 10 minutes. Serve.

Milk with White Poppy Seeds

Serves 1

10 saffron threads
1 cup milk
1 tablespoon white poppy seeds, soaked overnight in water to cover
1 tablespoon ghee
sucanot, to taste
seeds of 1 green cardamom pod, freshly ground
dash of freshly ground black pepper

In a nonporous mortar, grind the saffron threads until powdered. Stir in 3 tablespoons of the milk.

Drain the poppy seeds and grind to a fine paste in a mortar or electric grinder.

In a heavy pan, heat the ghee. Sauté the poppy seed paste for 3 minutes. Add the remaining ¾ cup plus 1 tablespoon milk and simmer, stirring frequently, for 10 minutes.

Add the saffron paste, sucanot, cardamom, and pepper and serve hot. (If served cool or lukewarm, honey rather than sucanot can be added.)

Poppy Seed Drink

with Nuts and Figs

Serves 2

2 tablespoons white poppy seeds
3 almonds
7 raw cashews
2 medium-to-large dried figs
2 tablespoons ghee
2 cups water or milk
sucanot, to taste

Soak the poppy seeds and nuts overnight in water to cover; in a separate container, soak the figs overnight in water to cover.

Drain the seeds and nuts. Peel the almonds. Combine all of the soaked ingredients, including the fig soaking water, and grind together in a mortar or blender.

In a heavy saucepan, heat the ghee over medium heat. Add the fig and nut paste and sauté, stirring constantly, until the ghee surfaces, about 30 minutes. Add the water and sucanot and blend well.

Serve hot in a glass or bowl. This mixture makes a powerful breakfast drink. It provides substantial heat, energy, and nourishment on cold winter days.

Shikangibin

Serves 4

1 quart water
juice of 1 lemon
4 teaspoons jaggery or sucanot

Spice Mixture:
1 tablespoon unroasted ground cumin
1 tablespoon roasted ground cumin
4 to 6 whole cloves, ground
seeds of 2 black cardamom pods, ground
seeds of 2 green cardamom pods, ground
pinch of black salt

In a pitcher, combine the water, lemon juice, and jaggery.

Combine all of the spice mixture ingredients and mix well.

Pour the liquid into four 8-ounce glasses and sprinkle each with a pinch of the spice mixture. The spices not only add flavor but make the drink easier to digest.

Store the remaining spice mixture airtight in a glass jar. This drink is a favorite treat on hot summer days in India.

Ginger Tea with Milk

Serves 4

3 cups whole milk
12 whole black peppercorns
1 small piece (¹/₂ to 1 inch long) fresh ginger, thinly sliced
2 to 3 teaspoons black tea leaves
1 tablespoon sucanot

In a saucepan, bring the milk, peppercorns, and ginger to a boil. Remove from the heat as soon as bubbles start to rise. Stir in the tea leaves and sucanot. Allow tea to steep for a few minutes. Strain and serve.

This is a good cold weather drink. It is beneficial for conditions of excess mucus. If taken on cold days, it prevents diseases brought about by cold weather. It cures colds and coughs and also fever brought on by colds.

Chai with Green Cardamom

Serves 4

1 cup milk
2 cups water
1 tablespoon black tea leaves
1 tablespoon sucanot
seeds of 1 green cardamom pod, freshly ground

In a saucepan, bring the milk and water to a boil. Remove mixture from the heat as soon as bubbles start to rise. Stir in the tea leaves, sucanot, and cardamom. Cover and allow to steep for a few minutes. Adjust the sucanot to taste. Strain and serve.

Almond Milk

Serves 2

2 cups milk
10 to 14 almonds, soaked overnight in water to cover
1 tablespoon honey
pinch of ground cardamom
plain yogurt, to taste (optional)

Scald the milk; set aside to cool.

Strain and peel the almonds. Grind them, along with the honey and cardamom, into a paste in a mortar or blender. Add enough of the cooled milk to make a creamy drink. If yogurt is added as a variation, reduce the milk somewhat and add a little more honey.

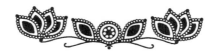

Appendix A

MENU COMBINATIONS

MENUS

Light Breakfasts

❖ Meusli
Vegetable Chips

❖ Mango Shake
Roasted Sunflower Seeds
Roasted Cashew Nuts

❖ Banana Cream with Rose Petals (or
any sweet fruit cream in season)
Mathris

❖ Halva with Carrots
Vegetable Chips

❖ Halva with Apple
Buckwheat Parathas with Green
Bananas
Mint Chutney

❖ Almond Milk
Mathris

❖ Yogurt with Saffron
Mathris or samosas

❖ Halva with Carrots
Kachoris

❖ Kheer with Carrots
Roasted Sunflower Seeds
Roasted Cashew Nuts

❖ Strawberry-Banana Cream
Dalia Khichari

❖ Plain Halva
Pappadams
Saunth with Tomatoes

❖ Magic Drink
Parathas

❖ Rabri with Pistachios and
Cardamom
Mathris

❖ Meusli
Mixed-Vegetable Pakoras

❖ Chai with Green Cardamom
Pappadams or Vegetable Chips

❖ Cracked Wheat with Dates,
Coconut, and Milk
Samosa and saunth

Snacks

- Mixed-Vegetable Pakora
  Mint Chutney or Pickled Garlic

- Potato with Cumin
  Parathas or chapatis

- Apple-Avocado-Banana Chutney
  Chapatis or mathris

- Mixed-Vegetable Pakora
  Saunth

- Rice and Urad Dal Pancakes
  Saunth

- Potatoes with Fenugreek
  Puris
  Saunth or pickles

- Potatoes with Cumin
  A mint or coriander chutney

- Asparagus Salad
  Parathas with potato or urad dal
  filling

- Carrot Salad
  Pappadams

- Moong Dal Khichari
  Raita with Potato and Tomato
  Pappadams

- Rice with Cumin
  Raita with Onion
  Pappadams

- Paneer with Onion
  Parathas, chapatis, or puris
  Saunth with Tomatoes

- Pulao with Peas
  Bean Ball in Yogurt (Dahi Balla)
  Pappadams

Main Meals

- Red Lentil Soup with Zucchini
  Green Peas with Potatoes
  Potato and Tomato Raita
  Chapatis, rice, or both

- Lentil Kababs
  Baked Potatoes with Raw Condi-
  ments (chokha)
  Saunth with Tomatoes
  Chapatis

- Red Cabbage with Mushrooms
  Zucchini with Cumin Seeds
  (soupy)
  Pickled Fruits and Vegetables
  Parathas

- Fried Paneer with Spinach
  Potatoes with Dried Fenugreek
  Puris or Potato Kachoris
  Saunth

- Broccoli Stems with Potatoes and
  Rice Paste
  Red Beets with Peas
  Bean Balls in Yogurt (Dahi Balla)
  Parathas

- Urad Dal with Tarka
  Okra with Onions and Garlic
  Chick-pea Flour Ladoos
  Mint Chutney
  Parathas

- Whole Moong Bean with Spices
  Paneer with Green Beans
  Tomato-Orange Salad
  Halva with Carrots
  Puris

❖ Kathal Kofta
Coconut Rice
Saunth
Pappadams
Rabri with Pistachios and
    Cardamom

❖ Buttermilk Soup with Chick-pea
    Flour (*Kadhi*)
Coconut Rice
Mint Chutney
Pappadams

❖ Potato Soup with Cumin Seeds
Broccoli and Mushroom Curry
Chapatis
Yogurt with Saffron

❖ Mixed Dal Stew with Tarka
Sweet and Sour Bitter Melon
Parathas or chapatis
Kheer with Poppy Seed

❖ Green Beans with Potatoes
Eggplant Bharta
Parathas with potato filling
Saunth
Kheer with Papaya

❖ Cauliflower with Carrots and Peas
Eggplant Purée
Pickled Fruits and Vegetables
Puris
Halva with Carrots

❖ Paneer with Red Beets and Peas
Stuffed parathas
Mint Chutney
Banana Sweet Cream with Rose
    Petals

❖ Okra with Onions and Garlic
Boiled Arwi Root (Taro)
Tomato-Orange Salad
Chapatis

❖ Cabbage Purée
Mushrooms and Onions
Parathas
Paneer with Saffron Ladoos

❖ Sweet-and-Sour Pumpkin
Celery with Potatoes and
    Fenugreek
Coriander Chutney
Chapatis
Ladoos with Moong Beans

❖ Turnips with Onions
Spinach with Mushrooms and
    Potatoes
Stuffed parathas
Tomato-Orange Salad
Ladoos with Cream of Wheat and
    Wheat Germ

❖ Potatoes with Onions and Yogurt
Leeks with Minced Vegetables
Chapatis
Halva with Apple

❖ Arwi Root (Taro) with Yogurt
Zucchini with Cumin seeds
Chapatis
Saunth
Rabri with Pistachios and Carda-
    mom

❖ Black Chick-peas with Ajwain
Red Cabbage with Mushrooms
Raita with Tomatoes and Potatoes
Puris
Date Ladoos

❖ Katras with Red Lentils
Pumpkin with Onion and Garlic
Parathas
Paneer Ladoos with Saffron

❖ Okra with Onions and Garlic
Boiled Plantains
Puris
Saunth
Papaya Sweet Cream

❖ Moong Dal Kichiari
Mint Chutney
Pappadams
Ladoos with Moong Beans

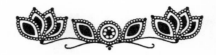

Appendix B

RECIPES FOR CHILDREN AND THE ELDERLY

Toastbread with Saffron Malai

Serves 1 to 2

Malai refers to the foam or crust that forms on boiled milk.

> ¹/₄ teaspoon saffron threads
> 3 tablespoons water
> 2 cups milk
> 2¹/₂ tablespoons brown sugar
> 1 tablespoon ghee (per toast)
> 1 slice whole wheat bread
> 1 teaspoon shredded pistachio nuts or rose petals, for decoration

Soak the saffron threads in the water for 3 hours.

To make the *malai*, cook the milk, uncovered, over extremely low heat very slowly, 1 to 2 hours, until you have 1¹/₂ cups of malai and ¹/₂ cup of milk remaining.

Dissolve the soaked saffron threads in the water with your fingers or in a mortar. Add 1 tablespoon of the saffron solution and 1 tablespoon of the sugar to the ¹/₂ cup milk. Pour the mixture into a wide, flat bowl. Add the remaining saffron and sugar to the malai.

In a flat chapati pan or griddle, heat the ghee over medium heat. Lightly sauté the slice of bread until toasted. Turn and add the remaining ghee.

Remove from pan and soak the toast in the saffron-milk mixture. Spread the saffron malai on top of the toast. Cool and decorate with pistachios or rose petals.

Serve with nuts, seeds, or any salty snack.

Paratha Soaked in Milk

Serves 1

1 cooked paratha (pages 205–206)
1 cup warm milk
1 teaspoon sucanot
pinch of ground green cardamom seeds or 1 tablespoon powdered
    coconut

Break the cooked paratha into small pieces and place in a bowl. Add all of
the remaining ingredients.

Serve for breakfast with salted seeds or nuts.

Halva with Cream of Wheat

Serves 4

1 cup Cream of Wheat
1 tablespoon ghee
3 cups water
½ cup jaggery or date sugar
½ cup mixed nuts, such as almonds, pine nuts, walnuts, etc., soaked,
    peeled, and ground into a paste
½ cup powdered coconut
seeds of 4 green cardamom pods, finely ground
freshly ground black pepper

In a nonstick frying pan, dry-roast the Cream of Wheat over low heat, stirring constantly. When the color changes, add the ghee and sauté for 2 minutes. Add the water and bring to a boil. Reduce the heat and stir in the jaggery.
Cook for 3 minutes and remove from the heat.

Stir in the nut paste and coconut powder. Allow to cool to lukewarm.
Stir in the fresh cardamom.

Stir and serve while still warm, with a sprinkling of black pepper.

Suji Kheer with Cream of Wheat

Serves 4

When preparing kheer, grind the cardamom just before adding it to the dish. Almonds, raisins, and dates served in this way give strength, stamina, and vigor to the elderly.

> 1 cup Cream of Wheat
> 3 cups hot water
> 8 pitted dates
> 1½ cups fresh milk
> 2 tablespoons raisins
> 20 almonds, soaked, peeled, and ground into paste
> 2 tablespoons powdered coconut
> seeds of 4 green cardamom pods, freshly ground

In a nonstick frying pan, dry-roast the Cream of Wheat over low heat, stirring constantly. When the wheat changes color, add the hot water and bring to a boil. Reduce the heat and add the dates; cook for 3 minutes. Add the milk and bring just to the boiling point; remove from the heat.

Stir in the raisins, almond paste, and coconut powder. Cool until lukewarm and stir in the fresh cardamom.

Stir and serve.

Appendix C

ABOUT MILK

TYPES OF COW'S MILK

In general, milk from a black cow is highly praised and recommended. It is said that such milk is nectar; it relieves Wind, Mucus, and Bile. It also relieves burning sensations, depression, heart disease, stomach troubles, kidney disorders, pain, jaundice, tuberculosis, anemia, pain from miscarriages, diseases of the uterus, chest troubles, and fatigue caused by overwork.

Milk from a spotted brown or red cow cures problems of the Bile. Milk from a yellow cow increases coughing, while that from a cow whose calf is dead creates Mucus, Bile and Wind. Also, milk from a cow that has stopped feeding her calf before the calf is four months old is strengthening but hard to digest.

The milk from a young cow is sweet, like elixir, and cures disorders created by Wind, Bile, and Mucus. That of an old cow, or one over three months pregnant, increases Bile; it is dehydrating and creates irritation in the throat: This milk is not recommended. If it is not boiled within three hours of being drawn, the milk becomes heavy and creates Wind, Bile, and Mucus.

Hot milk cures diseases caused by excess Bile (Pitta) and excess Mucus (Kapha). Cold milk is strengthening but increases Mucus. It is hard to digest and also slightly constipating.

OTHER TYPES OF MILK

Goat's milk is easy to digest. It cures diseases of the kidneys and urinary tract, especially when the urine is deep yellow or reddish. For diseases caused by heat or for weak digestive fire, coughs, colds, and tuberculosis, goat's milk is a food and a medicine.

Sheep's milk has a salty taste. It has less fat than cow's milk and cures disease of the kidneys and urinary tract. This milk thickens and increases semen; it is also an aphrodisiac.

Camel's milk is sour. It can be stored only after being boiled. It cures tuberculosis, pneumonia, and skin diseases, as well as Mucus and urinary troubles.

Elephant's milk is unctuous, heavy, and hard to digest, but it is the most powerful of all milks. It increases sensuality and virility if used regularly over a long period. Applied topically, it cures eye troubles.

Donkey's milk is cold, light, and unctuous. It helps cure excess heat in the body. It cures syphilis, pleurisy, and all diseases of the chest region. Before either the smallpox or chicken pox season starts, Indian mothers try to give their children a small amount of donkey's milk to prevent these diseases. The donkey is the vehicle of the goddess Shitla—the goddess of smallpox.

Horse's milk is a superior medicine for healing mental disorders and schizophrenia, especially if the madness is prompted by excessive heat or occurs during the hot season. It is also beneficial for patients with hysteria.

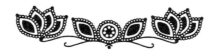

GLOSSARY OF INGREDIENTS

Ajwain: A spice seed used in North Indian cooking and in many of the recipes in this book. It is widely available at Indian and Middle Eastern groceries.

Arwi Root (Taro): A root vegetable that can vary tremendously in size. As used in the recipes in this book, a small, medium, or large arwi root should be equivalent in size to a small, medium, or large potato. (See also Foods and Their Healing Properties, page 32.)

Asafoetida (Hing): See Foods and Their Healing Properties, page 38.

Basmati Rice: A long-grain scented rice originally cultivated in India and now used in rice dishes throughout the world. All the rice dishes in this book call for unpolished white Basmati rice. If you use brown Basmati, you will need to slightly increase the cooking time. Available at health food stores as well as Indian and specialty groceries.

Bitter Melon (Karela): See Foods and Their Healing Properties, page 33.

Black Cumin Seeds: See Foods and Their Healing Properties, page 43.

Black Salt: Reddish-gray in color, this salt contains valuable trace minerals and iron. It is used in the recipes in this book for its healthful properties as well as its distinctive flavor. It is not interchangeable with white salt.

Bottle Gourd Squash (Louki): A delicious Indian summer squash. Available fresh at Indian groceries and at Asian groceries where it is known as *hula*.

Chapati Flour: A type of low-gluten wheat flour especially suited to flat breads. Available at Indian and Middle Eastern groceries.

Coconut, dried: The recipes in this book call for dried coconut in several forms. Unless otherwise indicated, feel free to use the grated, ground, flaked, and powdered forms interchangeably, depending upon what is available to you at health food stores or Indian and specialty groceries.

Fenugreek Leaves (Methi), dried: A bitter herb that is difficult to obtain fresh unless it is home-grown. The dried leaves (follow recipe instructions for soaking) are readily available at Indian groceries.

Ghee: See Foods and Their Healing Properties, page 23 and Ghee and Oils, page 73.

Gur: See Foods and Their Healing Properties, page 48.

Jackfruit: A tropical fruit that is treated more like a vegetable in Indian cooking. The recipes in this book call for fresh, but canned may also be used. It is not necessary to steam the canned fruit before mashing it into a paste. Available at Indian groceries.

Jaggery (Gur): See Foods and Their Healing Properties, page 48.

Karela: See Bitter Melon.

Kela (Plantain): See Foods and Their Healing Properties, pages 34-35.

Louki: See Bottle Gourd Squash.

Lotus Root, fresh: The underground rhizome of the lotus plant, used as a vegetable in Indian cooking. Available at Asian groceries.

Mango Powder: Used for its sour flavor. Available at Indian groceries.

Mustard Oil: Deliciously pungent, this oil is cleansing to the stomach and intestinal walls. It should always be consumed in its raw state, uncooked. (See also Ghee and Oils, page 73.)

Okra, dried: The dried pods of the okra plant. Available at Middle Eastern groceries.

Plantain: See Kela.

Pomegranate Seeds, dried: See Foods and Their Healing Properties, page 45.

Rock Sugar: Sugar in crystal form, popular in India and available at Indian groceries.

Rose Petal Jam: A specialty condiment available at Indian groceries.

Saffron: Sold in powder form and in threads (a pinch of saffron is approximately equal to ten to twelve threads), this spice is costly and is easily adulterated in the powdered form. The threads are usually soaked and ground before they are added to foods. Ask for threads or high quality powder at Indian, Middle Eastern, or specialty groceries. (See also Foods and Their Healing Properties, pages 45-46.)

Silver Leaf: Silver in the form of a paper-thin, edible foil that is used to decorate sweets. Available at Indian groceries.

Soy Yogurt: Made from soy milk, this yogurt is very good for those who cannot tolerate dairy products in their diet. Available at health food stores.

Suran (Zaminkand, Indian Yam): An Indian root vegetable that is reddish-orange inside. It is cooked with sour-tasting ingredients to neutralize its natural astringency. Available canned and sometimes fresh at Indian groceries.

Tamarind Pulp: Used as an ingredient in certain dishes to impart a sour taste. You may substitute dried pomegranate seeds (3 tablespoons for every tablespoon tamarind) or mango powder (1 1/2 tablespoons for every tablespoon tamarind). Prepared tamarind pulp is available at Indian groceries. See also Foods and Their Healing Properties, page 46.

Taro Root: See Arwi.

Tinda: Small, apple-shaped green squash. Other gourd-type squashes can be used in its place. Available at Indian groceries—fresh in late summer and canned year-round.

SOURCES OF SUPPLY

The following suppliers will provide Indian spices and other ingredients by mail. Write or call for catalogs and mail order information.

California

Bazaar of India
1810 University
Berkeley, CA 94703
(510) 548-4110

India Sweets and Spices
9409 Venice Boulevard
Los Angeles, CA 90230
(310) 837-5286

Florida

Indian Grocery Store
2342 Douglas Road
Coral Gables, FL 33134
(305) 448-5869

Missouri

Seema Enterprises
10616 Page Avenue
St. Louis, MO 63132
(314) 423-9990

New York

Annapurna
127 East 28th Street
New York, NY 10016
(212) 889-7540

Kalustyan's
123 Lexington Avenue
New York, NY 10016
(212) 685-3451

Little India Stores, Inc.
128 East 28th Street
New York, NY 10016
(212) 683-1619

Spice Corner
135 Lexington Avenue
New York, NY 10016
(212) 689-5182

Ohio
    Indian Cafe and Grocery
    5230 Bethel Center Mall
    Columbus, OH 43220
    (614) 451-8121

Pennsylvania
    House of Spices
    4101 Walnut Street
    Philadelphia, PA 19104
    (215) 222-1111

Vermont
    The Herb Closet
    104 Main Street
    Montpelier, VT 05602
    (802) 223-0888
Full line of Ayurvedic herbs and
formulas

Wisconsin
    India Groceries and Spices
    10633 West North Avenue
    Wauwatosa, WI 53226
    (414) 771-3535

Canada
    Daya Health Food
    8236 Yonge Street
    Horn Hill, Ontario
    L4J 1W6 Canada
    (905) 881-0454

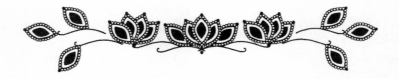

INDEX

Note: Recipe titles are capitalized and are listed after general information in the entries.